Earl Mindell's

HERB BIBLE

EARL MINDELL, R.Ph., Ph.D.

A FIRESIDE BOOK
PUBLISHED BY SIMON & SCHUSTER
NEW YORK LONDON TORONTO SYDNEY TOKYO SINGAPORE

The ideas, procedures, and suggestions contained in this book are not intended to replace the services of a trained health professional. All matters regarding your health require medical supervision. You should consult your physician before adopting the procedures in this book. Any applications of the treatments set forth in this book are at the reader's discretion.

Simon & Schuster/Fireside
Simon & Schuster Building
Rockefeller Center
1230 Avenue of the Americas
New York, New York 10020

SIMON & SCHUSTER, FIRESIDE, and colophon
are registered trademarks of Simon & Schuster Inc.

Manufactured in the United States of America

10 9 8 7 6 5 4 3 2 1
10 9 8 7   PBK

Library of Congress Cataloging-in-Publication Data

Mindell, Earl.
[Herb bible]
Earl Mindell's herb bible / Earl L. Mindell.
p.   cm.
Includes bibliographical references and index.
1. Herbs—Therapeutic use.   I. Title. II. Title: Herb bible.
RM666.H33M56 1992
615'.321—dc20   91-18798
                                                             CIP

ISBN 0-671-76113-7
0-671-76122-6 (pbk)

This book is dedicated to Gail, Alannah, Evan, my parents and family, my friends and associates, and to the continuing happiness and health of people everywhere.

Acknowledgments

I wish to express my deep and lasting appreciation to my friends and associates who have assisted me in the preparation of this book, especially: J. Kenney, Ph.D.; Linus Pauling, Ph.D.; Harold Segal, Ph.D.; Bernard Bubman, R.Ph.; Mel Rich, R.Ph.; Sal Messineo, Pharm.D., R.Ph.; Arnold Fox, M.D.; Dennis Huddleson, M.D.; Stewart Fisher, M.D.; the late Robert Mendselsohn, M.D.; Gershon Lesser, M.D.; David Velkoff, M.D.; Rory Jaffee, M.D.; Vicki Hufnagel, M.D.; Donald Cruden, O.D.; Joel Strom, D.D.S.; Nathan Sperling, D.D.S. A special thanks to Rob McCaleb of the Herb Research Foundation for his assistance. I would also like to thank Carol Colman Gerber and my editor, Toni Sciarra, for their help with this project. A special thanks to my agent, Richard Curtis, for his support throughout the years. Finally, I would like to express my gratitude to the Dominion Herbal College where I received my degree as a chartered herbalist on July 30, 1984.

Contents

Before You Begin This Book   11

1. What Is An Herb?   19

2. The "Hot Hundred"   33

3. Traditional Favorites   175

4. Herbs from Around the World   189

5. The Herbal Medicine Cabinet   215

6. A Woman's Body   227

7. A Man's Body   239

8. Herbal Preventive Medicine   245

9. Looking Good   255

10. Aromatherapy   265

CONTENTS

Resources   271

Bibliography   277

Index   285

Before You Begin This Book

I started pharmacy school in 1958, just as the pill-popping era was dawning. By the time I graduated and entered practice, there seemed to be a pill for whatever ailed us. Have a sore throat? Take an antibiotic. Think a headache is coming on? Reach for an aspirin. Need to drop some weight or pick up some energy? Try amphetamines. Want to calm down? A tranquilizer will help you relax. This was also the dawn of the space age. We were preparing to send a man to the moon in a space capsule. Thus it was only logical for us to believe that we would soon be able to cure the common cold, flu, acne, and various catastrophic illnesses with time-release capsules. The notion that lifestyle, diet, or exercise could possibly influence health was considered unscientific and profoundly silly. "Scientific" remedies were not hard to find, however. They were widely advertised and came packaged in attractive boxes, bottles, or blister packs. Natural remedies—the kind our grandmothers and great-grandmothers relied on—were dismissed as pure hokum. These were the days when there seemed to be nothing that nature could do that humans could not do better.

Against this backdrop, I reluctantly—very reluctantly—registered for the required course in pharmacognosy, the study of drugs derived from plants. My classmates and I disparagingly called the course "weeds and seeds," and we thought that it was utterly weird. We went on field trips and foraged for plants known for their medicinal value. With my own hands, I picked them, dried them, and with an old-fashioned mortar and pestle, turned them into useful drugs. In the process, my skepticism about so-called natural remedies began to fade and I started studying the literature—some might call it lore—of natural remedies. I was astonished to discover that people have been using natural remedies for thousands of years to treat—and treat successfully—a wide variety of ills, ranging from heartburn to heart disease. In fact, prior to World War II, herbal medications were listed side-by-side with chemical drugs in the *U.S. Pharmacopeia*, the official listing of accepted medicines. Even today, nearly 50 percent of the thousands of drugs commonly used and prescribed are either derived from a plant source or contain chemical imitations of a plant compound. The list is impressive:

Digitalis, a potent cardiotonic, is derived from the foxglove plant.

Aspirin is a chemical imitation of salicin from the bark of the white willow tree.

Reserpine, a blood pressure medicine, is actually an ancient Indian remedy derived from an Asian shrub.

Ephedrine and pseudoephedrine, found in many over-the-counter cold remedies, are derived from the ephedra plant, which has been used in China to treat colds and flu for more than five thousand years!

Quinine, a famous malaria treatment, and quinidine, an antiarrhythmic medication, are made from the bark of the cinchona tree.

Vincritisine and vinblastine, two of our most success-
ful cancer treatments, are derived from the rosy periwinkle tree, which is native to southern Madagascar.
Medicine derived from this plant has saved the lives
of thousands of victims of childhood leukemia.

Penicillin, the grandfather of antibiotics, is actually a
mold, an organism produced by a fungus, a primitive
plant.

Thus, I owe my lifelong interest in herbal medicine to
the course called Pharmacognosy 101. After graduation, I
began collecting antique herbal guides (often called "herbals"), some of which are more than two centuries old. But
I never took my herbals to the pharmacy with me, because
herbalism was considered obsolete. Indeed, not long after
I graduated, pharmacognosy was dropped from the list of
required courses by many pharmacy schools. (Ironically,
today many schools have reintroduced the course and
many others are considering it.)

The major reason for the decline in herbalism was not
the herbs' efficacy but economics. Herbs are not profitable.
In the United States, most herbs are not recognized as
drugs or as having any medicinal value. Rather, they are
classified as food or food additives. Even if an herb is
known to be beneficial as a medicine, it cannot be sold as
a drug until it receives the official stamp of approval by the
Food and Drug Administration, and approval does not
come quickly, easily, or cheaply. Where the introduction
of new drugs is concerned, the United States is one of the
most restrictive countries in the world. The extensive test-
ing required to achieve official drug status—that is, to
prove a substance is safe and effective—can cost tens of
millions of dollars and take many years. (This explains
why the cost of the average prescription has risen tenfold
since 1950!)

Moreover, natural substances cannot be patented.

When a pharmaceutical company creates a new drug, the company is given a seventeen-year exclusive right to market that product so that the company can recoup its research and development costs. Were a pharmaceutical company to simply package an herb, the company would receive no such market protection. Thus, there is little incentive to spend time and money investigating the potential benefits of an herb that people can grow themselves or that competitors are free to market. It's not surprising, therefore, that many pharmaceutical houses have lost interest in pursuing plant drugs altogether and instead have focused their research and development efforts on new synthetic medications. An unfortunate consequence of this shift in emphasis to synthetic drugs was that many time-honored natural remedies were displaced and, at least for a while, were forgotten.

Today, however, we are witnessing a renewed interest in herbal remedies, not only on the part of whole-earth advocates but from solid medical practitioner types as well. One reason is the recognition that although synthetic drugs have certainly performed many miracles and saved countless lives, they have not turned out to be the "silver bullet" that pharmacologists hoped they would be. Virtually all of these drugs have well-known side effects ranging from the unpleasant to the lethal. In many cases, they are not even effective. For example, antibiotics, for all their ability to defeat bacterial infections, are essentially useless against viruses, and many of the diseases that plague us today—from the Shanghai flu to AIDS to chronic fatigue syndrome—are viral syndromes.

Another reason for the growing interest in herbal remedies is that we now know that many over-the-counter medications can be hazardous. For example, many consumers turned to acetaminophen as a "safe alternative" to aspirin because they feared that aspirin would irritate stomachs or lead to Reye's syndrome in children. Recently, acetaminophen has been linked to kidney damage. Antacids, among the most widely used over-the-counter drugs, can actually cause stomach irritation. As every cold or allergy sufferer knows, many popular antihistamines cause drowsiness or excitability, and trigger a "rebound effect" resulting in more congestion.

Perhaps the major reason for our renewed interest in herbalism can be attributed to the new emphasis on preventive medicine. The pendulum of science is on its return swing, and we now know that lifestyle and nutrition play significant roles in averting disease. There is a growing recognition that herbs, too, can play a vital role in promoting wellness. Unlike drugs, many herbs are taken as "tonics," that is, like many vitamins, they can be used primarily to maintain good health. Studies show that there are herbs that can reduce cholesterol, improve circulation, and even prevent cancer. Some herbs have been shown to enhance immune function, thus helping the body to fight against disease. Obviously, most of us would prefer to take an herb that would help us stay healthy than a drug when we are sick!

Even as we in the United States were moving away from natural remedies, herbs were being studied and used very successfully abroad. Foreign medical journals are filled with reports of plant drugs found to be useful in treating cancer, heart disease, and other serious ailments. In countries such as England, Germany, France, China, and Japan, herbs are recognized as valid remedies and are often incorporated in conventional medical treatment. In West Germany, for instance, a doctor may prescribe the herb valerian for cases of mild anxiety and the patent drug Valium when a stronger drug is needed. Throughout Europe, herbal remedies and over-the-counter drugs are sold side-by-side. A British cold sufferer can choose between a packaged herbal cold remedy and a conventional cold capsule.

In health food stores, herb shops, and even in many

drugstores around the United States, we are beginning to see prepackaged herbal remedies similar to those that are so popular in Europe. Go into a drugstore or health food store and you are likely to find packages of ginkgo capsules and ginseng extract next to the vitamins and cold medications. In the United States, however, herbs are not recognized as drugs, and manufacturers are not allowed to make therapeutic claims for their products. Therefore, labeling is often vague. This is not a problem for people who are familiar with herbal medicine, but it can be very frustrating for people who are not. Unfortunately, there are few places to go for information. Your local pharmacist probably can't answer your questions, because chances are, he never took a course in pharmacognosy. Most doctors know little about herbs. The village shaman—the traditional medicine man or woman—has gone the way of the milkman.

Standard herb guides tend to be quite detailed and eclectic because they were geared to people who have the time and space to grow, dry, and prepare their own remedies, and who are able to decode the jargon typical of old-fashioned herbals. I've written the *Herb Bible* to help close this information gap. Here, I might interject that educating people about alternative approaches to healthcare is something that I have enjoyed doing for many years. In 1979, I wrote *Earl Mindell's Vitamin Bible*, which is still widely read today and is generally regarded as one of the books that helped to popularize vitamin use in the United States. When I first wrote the *Vitamin Bible*, vitamins were viewed as being "for health and food types only," and health food stores were about the only place where you could buy anything more "exotic" than one-a-day–type vitamins. Today, vitamins are sold everywhere, from the corner drugstore to fashionable department stores. I think that in terms of public acceptance, herbs are where vitamins were ten years ago.

The *Herb Bible* has a similar mission to that of the *Vitamin*

Bible in that it is geared to the novice who is interested in exploring the world of herbal remedies. I write about herbs that are easily available in most herb shops and health stores and that are also easy to use.

In the first chapter, I explain exactly what herbs are, how they work, and how to buy them. I have assessed the hundreds of herbs in use in the United States and have compiled a list of what I call the "Hot Hundred." It appears in chapter 2. These are herbs that are becoming popular because they are particularly useful for the kinds of ailments that afflict modern men and women. I describe exactly what each herb does and how to use it.

"Traditional Favorites," a selection of time-honored herbal remedies that are still popular today, are reviewed in chapter 3. In chapter 4, "Herbs from Around the World," you will learn about age-old remedies from China, India, South America, and those used by Native Americans in the United States. "The Herbal Medicine Cabinet," in chapter 5, will tell you about the herbs that no household should be without.

Chapter 6, "A Woman's Body," deals with problems that affect women and explains how herbs can provide significant relief. Chapter 7, "A Man's Body," offers herbal solutions to common problems that afflict men, from premature baldness to prostate trouble.

"Herbal Preventive Medicine," in chapter 8, examines how herbs may be used to prevent heart diseases, cancer, and other ailments. In chapter 9, "Looking Good," I discuss herbal personal grooming products that can be used by both sexes. "Aromatherapy," the increasingly widespread practice of using scented oils for healing, is covered in chapter 10.

The Resources section explains how to find an herbally oriented physician and where to obtain more information on herbs. It also provides a partial listing of mail-order companies that sell herbal products.

Herbal medicine is not a panacea for all of our ills—there

is no substitution for a healthy lifestyle. Prevention is still the best medicine and, in my opinion, always will be. There are times, however, when conventional medicine is absolutely essential. Anyone who has ever been treated successfully with a synthetic drug—who had a strep infection that did not develop into rheumatic fever thanks to amoxicillin or who beat cancer thanks to chemotherapy— owes a debt of gratitude to the pharmaceutical houses that developed these drugs. There should be room, however, for a wide variety of treatment options, and I believe that herbal medicine deserves a place high on that list.

This book does not encourage the self-diagnosis and treatment of disease. If you are seriously ill, you should receive proper medical attention. There are many situations, however, in which it may be appropriate to self-medicate. Few of us call the doctor every time we get a headache, develop a cold, get indigestion, suffer menstrual cramps, or experience the aches and pains of mild arthritis. Most of us rely on over-the-counter medications to treat these benign problems. This book will show you how to select and use natural herbal remedies for these everyday problems. If the problems become severe or persist for more than a week, I feel it is advisable to call your physician.

Important: If you are now taking any drugs—either over-the-counter or prescription—or have any medical conditions or problems, it is wise to consult a naturally oriented physician who is aware of herb–drug interactions and any potentially dangerous side effects before taking any herbal remedies.

CHAPTER 1

What Is An Herb?

The term *herb* has usually been used to refer to any plant or plant part valued for its medicinal, savory, or aromatic qualities. For the purposes of this book, herb means any plant that is primarily used for medicinal purposes.

There are approximately 380,000 species of plants on earth that we have identified and several hundred thousand that have yet to be discovered. (Right now, many scientists are desperately trying to catalogue the plants in the Amazon rainforest in the belief that there are thousands of potential plant cures that are rapidly being destroyed by development.) Out of the number of known plants, about 260,000 are classified as higher plants, which means that they contain chlorophyll and perform a process called *photosynthesis*. In photosynthesis, plants utilize the energy provided by sunlight to manufacture carbohydrates from carbon dioxide and water. All the members of the higher plant group have the potential to offer medical benefits. Only 10 percent, however, have actually been studied for this purpose.

In the *Herb Bible*, I refer to each herb by its two names: the familiar name by which it is commonly known and a Latin botanical name describing its genus and species. The genus or first name is the general grouping of plants by family. Although plants in a given genus are not identical, they have in common certain similar characteristics. The species is a more specific way of defining each plant's distinctive qualities. For example, onions, garlic, and chive are all members of the *Allium* genus. However, each of these herbs is classified as a different species.

HOW DO HERBS WORK?

The living cells of plants can be likened to miniature chemical factories. They take in raw materials—carbon dioxide, water, and sunlight—and convert them into useful nutrients. Oxygen is a by-product of this process. Many herbs are rich in compounds that are pharmacologically active, that is, they exert a profound effect on certain animal tissues and organs. Therefore, they can be used as drugs in treating, curing, or preventing disease. A plant may consist of several components including leaves, roots, fruit, flowers, bark, stems, or seeds. Any of these parts may contain the active ingredients that give the plant its medicinal properties.

The herbal pharmacy is a rich one. There are herbs that target specific organ systems and there are herbs that are used as general tonics to promote overall health. There are herbs that soothe pain and inflammation, and still other herbs that work to reduce muscle spasm. Some herbs have a stimulating effect; others have a relaxing effect. Some kill bacteria; others activate the body's own immune system so that it can ward off invading organisms.

Thousands of years ago, when people first began using herbs, they had no idea why herbs worked. All they knew was that a certain plant elicited a desired result. When our ancestors first used foxglove to treat heart failure, they didn't know that this fuchsia-flowered plant contained molecules called glycosides that stimulate heart cells. When mothers in the Middle Ages soothed a scraped knee with a comfrey leaf, they didn't know that the plant's astringent tannins formed a protective surface over the wound, thus promoting healing. When Chinese healers prescribed licorice for arthritis flare-ups, they didn't know that it contained saponins, antiinflammatory compounds similar to natural steroid hormones. When the Ancient Egyptians fed garlic to their slaves to keep them healthy, they didn't know that it contained volatile oils that fight infection.

Thanks to modern laboratory techniques, we now understand how many of these herbs function. We are able to break down each plant into its basic molecular structure and analyze its extracts. Although we know a great deal more than our ancestors did about how some herbs work, there are still many more that need to be researched. Ironically, due to the lack of scientific data for many herbs, we must still rely heavily on information transmitted through folklore, antique herbals, and word-of-mouth.

Caution!

Just because herbs are natural substances doesn't mean that they can be used indiscriminately. Herbs can be strong medicine. Before trying any herbal remedy, be sure that you know what it does, how to use it, and the possible side effects. Never exceed the recommended dose. As a general rule, few medical problems occur from ingesting herbal remedies, but the potential for an allergic or toxic reaction is always there. In addition, about 1 percent of all plants are poisonous. Therefore, I do not recommend that people gather their own herbs unless they are skilled botanists. Pregnant women should take herbs only under the direction of a knowledgeable physician or midwife. Parents should check with a qualified healthcare practitioner before giving herbs to children.

THE FIRST "WONDER DRUG"

The Ebers Papyrus, named after Egyptologist Georg Ebers, is a papyrus written around 1600 B.C. that refers to more than seven hundred plant medicines including peppermint, myrrh, and castor oil. This early medical text recommends applying a moldy piece of bread to open wounds. In 1928—thousands of years later—by pure happenstance, Sir Alexander Fleming noticed in his laboratory that bread mold was a potent antibiotic. His observation led to the development of penicillin and spawned the era of the "wonder drugs."

HOW TO BUY HERBS

In the past, if you wanted to use an herbal remedy, you had two choices: You could either grow your own or try to find it in the woods. And that was just the beginning of your labor. Once you found it, you had to pick it, dry it, grind it, boil it, or mix it in an alcohol solution to create a potent remedy. Needless to say, the process was extremely time consuming. In addition, due to differences in climate and growing conditions, you could never be absolutely sure that the plant you picked contained enough of the right active ingredients or that you had processed it in just the right way.

Today, you don't have to be a gardener or a chemist to use herbs safely and effectively. Similar to vitamins, herbs are now widely available in health food stores and herb shops. They are packaged in easy-to-use forms that eliminate much of the work and the guesswork. Several of the companies that have been making and selling vitamins for years now have their own lines of herb products and offer a standardized, guaranteed potency product. This means that herbs sold by these and other reputable companies contain uniform levels of the compound (or compounds) believed to be responsible for the plant's medicinal activity. Not all herbs are available in this form, but when they are, I feel they are preferable to nonstandardized products. In addition, some companies are now offering fresh, freeze-dried herbs that may preserve more of the herb's active ingredients than traditional processing methods. In some cases, I advise using the freeze-dried herb if it is available.

Because of the concern over pesticides and processing techniques, many manufacturers offer organically grown, nonirradiated products. There are times in the *Herb Bible* when I will recommend fresh herbs, but only in cases where they are easily accessible. In most cases, however, I recommend using a commercial herbal preparation.

Is it better to buy herbs in an herb shop than in a health food store? It all depends on what you're looking for. As a rule, herb shops generally carry a greater selection of dried herbs and teas, including many of the more exotic varieties. Although visiting an herb shop is a wonderful way to spend an afternoon, a well-stocked health food store may actually offer a better selection of prepared herbal remedies. If you don't live near an herb store or a health food store, or don't have time to shop, it is possible to buy herbs through the mail. (In the Resources section of the *Herb Bible*, you will find a partial list of mail-order companies that sell herbs.)

Here is a list of some of the different ways in which herbs are packaged and sold:

1. *Capsules and tablets.* Many of the more popular herbs are now sold in capsule and tablet form in various potencies. The usual dose, depending on the herb, is 2 to 3 tablets or capsules, taken 2 to 3 times daily. Always follow the directions provided on the label.

2. *Extracts or tinctures.* Extracts or tinctures are liquid herbal products typically prepared by soaking herbs in an alcohol solution. However, there are some new alcohol-free extracts on the market that may be preferable in certain instances, especially for diabetics, pregnant women, children, and other people who ought to avoid alcohol. The usual dose, depending on the herb, is 10 to 30 drops, 2 to 3 times daily. Use as directed. (Homeopathic extracts used by homeopathic practitioners are much stronger than conventional herbal tinctures and are strictly regulated by the FDA. They should be used only in conjunction with treatment by a homeopathic practitioner.)

3. *Powders.* Some herbs are sold in powdered form. The required dose may be mixed in water or juice. If the herb is bitter, a drop of honey may be used as a sweetener. Some people, however, may prefer the convenience of capsules. Most stores will sell empty capsules, usually in #0 size, that hold 400–450 mg of herb. Kosher, gelatin-free capsules are available for vegetarians and people on restricted, religious diets.

4. *Dried herbs.* Dried herbs are sold in bulk, usually in large glass bottles. They should be stored in an airtight container at home, out of direct sunlight. These herbs may be put into capsules, but are usually brewed into a tea. It's very easy to do. Simply put 1 heaping tablespoon of herb

into a tea ball and submerge it in 1 cup of hot water. Steep for 10 to 15 minutes. Drink the tea while it's hot. If you double the recipe, the leftover tea can be stored in the refrigerator and reheated. (If you don't use a tea ball, you can put the dried herb directly into the hot liquid. When the tea is brewed, strain the liquid before drinking it.)

5. *Prepared teas.* Many herbs these days are sold in tea bag form. Keep in mind that many of the teas you find in health food stores, especially those designated as "home remedies" for colds, are more potent than herbal tea sold in supermarkets and should only be used as directed.

6. *Juice.* Some herbs are sold in juice form. They should be used according to package directions.

7. *Combination herbal products.* A wide range of herbal remedies combining two or more herbs that work well together are available in capsule, tea, and extract form. For example, several herbs that are good for maintaining heart health, or herbs good for immune function, may be combined in one easy-to-use product. Use as directed.

8. *Creams and ointments.* Many herbs that are commonly used externally are now sold commercially as creams and ointments. These preparations can have potent ingredients and should be used only as directed.

9. *Essential oils.* These are primarily used for bath oils, perfumes, massage oils, and for aromatherapy, which is the practice of using certain fragrances to promote health and relaxation. Essential oils are for external use only.

10. *Personal care.* Several personal care product lines sell natural, pure, herbal products without any synthetic ingredients. These include herbal shampoos (*real* herbal

shampoos, not the herbal-scented shampoos you find in the supermarket), facial cleansers, deodorants, moisturizers, toothpaste, and even herbal mouthwash. There are also herbal cosmetic lines. These are excellent alternatives to chemical-laden products that can be potentially irritating for many people. An added plus is that many of these product lines are cruelty-free, that is, they are not tested on animals.

Shelf Life of Herbs

Dried herbs should be as fresh as possible. Try to buy them in a store with a good turnover. Some packaged herbal products will have an expiration date printed on the package that tells you when the herb is too stale to be useful. Unopened containers of tablets and capsules are usually good for up to two years. If opened, dispose of them after one year.

Be an Alert Consumer

Unfortunately, there have been several disturbing stories in the natural food industry press about unscrupulous manufacturers or retailers who use a minute quantity of a particular herb and then market the product as a true herbal remedy or they mislabel the product altogether. To ensure the quality of the product you are buying, purchase herbs sold by reputable companies that have been in the herb business for at least ten years. If you have questions about a particular product line, call the manufacturer. The reliable companies welcome consumer inquiries. Get to know the owner of your local health food store or herb shop, and don't be afraid to ask questions. If you're buying herbs in bulk, find out who is supplying the store. If you don't understand the ingredients in a particular product, ask the owner to explain. Most will be more than willing to share their knowledge and information with you.

HIPPOCRATES: THE FATHER OF MEDICINE

Historians know surprisingly little about the man who is revered as the "father of medicine." In fact, we're not even certain of the exact dates of his birth and death. All we know is that Hippocrates was born sometime in the fourth century B.C. on the Greek island of Kos. He died around 377 B.C. During his lifetime, he was a well-respected physician and teacher. Hippocrates rejected the idea that evil spirits were responsible for disease, the prevailing notion of the day. Rather, he proposed the radical theory that illness was a result of the improper balance of bodily fluids that he called the "four humors"—blood, phlegm, yellow bile, and black bile. According to Hippocrates, the real culprit was a poor diet, which left "residues" in the body. The father of medicine advocated the use of diet and plant medicines to prevent and cure disease. The Hippocratic oath, which doctors still take today, was probably composed by a follower of Hippocrates in the third century.

TAKING THE RIGHT AMOUNT

The amount of herb required for a desired result may vary from person to person, depending on a number of factors. For example, a heavy person may require a larger dose than a very thin person. An older adult usually requires a smaller dose than a younger one. Regardless of age or weight, a person who is highly responsive to medications may require only a small amount of herb. To accommodate these differences, the recommended daily dose usually allows for some flexibility. For example, if in the "Hot Hundred," I advise you to mix between 10 and 30 drops of herbal extract in a cup of liquid, *start with the lowest dose first* to test for any adverse reactions. If the herb agrees with you, you may gradually work your way up to the maximum dose, if need be. However, if you are taking an herb for a particular problem, such as arthritic pain, and you find relief with the lower dose, there's no reason to increase it. Be very careful not to exceed the recommended dosages stated on the labels. Also, be aware that some herbs should be taken only for brief periods of time for a particular problem—they are not safe for long-term use. Make sure that you learn as much as possible about any herb before taking it.

THE BEST TIME TO TAKE HERBAL REMEDIES

Some people may feel nauseous if they take herbs on an empty stomach. If you use herbs on a daily basis, wait until after meals to take them. If you're using an herb for a specific problem, such as menstrual cramps or headache, take the herb as needed.

Use your common sense: Don't take a stimulating herb at night when you want to wind down. Don't take an herb that makes you sleepy before going to work or driving.

A BRIEF HISTORY OF HERBAL MEDICINE

The practice of herbal medicine may predate the human race. Animal behaviorists have observed that many animals instinctively seek specific plants when they are sick.

As anyone who has ever cared for a dog knows, when the animal grazes on grass, it means that he probably has a stomachache. Early humans may have learned about the healing power of plants by mimicking this kind of animal behavior.

The first "herbal guide" dates back five thousand years to the Sumerians, who used herbs such as caraway and thyme for healing. Ayurveda, the traditional medicine of India that is still practiced today, may be even older. Herbal prescriptions were written in hieroglyphics on papyrus in Ancient Egypt. Onions and garlic were favorite remedies. The first Chinese herbal, the *Wu Shi Er Bing Fang* (*Prescriptions for Fifty-two Diseases*) was compiled somewhere between 1065 B.C. and 711 B.C. It included herbs such as licorice, ginger, and astragalus root (which are all listed in the Hot Hundred!) The Bible is full of references to herbs such as aloe, myrrh, and frankincense.

The Greek physician Hippocrates (460–377 B.C.), who is believed to be the first practicing physician, recorded between three hundred and four hundred plant remedies in his writings. In the first century, another Greek physician, Dioscorides, listed five hundred plant medicines in his herbal, *De Materia Medica*, which was used until the seventeenth century. Galen (A.D. 137), a famous physician who ministered to a Roman emperor and his gladiators, used a blend of herbs and magic to cure patients.

During the Middle Ages, ancient herbal remedies were passed on from generation to generation, but there was no uniform system of healing. A woman with a gynecological problem might seek help from the village "wise woman" who had learned the art of herbal healing from another woman. The more affluent might seek care from a doctor who would prescribe his own homemade concoction made from plant or animal parts. Although the church emphasized faith healing over other forms of healing, local monks preserved many of the early Greek and Roman medical texts. Many monasteries grew their own herbs and used them to treat their parishioners.

In the fifteenth century, the development of the printing press made information more accessible to the masses. John Gerard, a physician to the Tudor family, published *The Herball or General Historie of Plantes* in 1597, one of the first English herbals. It was quickly followed by Nicholas Culpeper's *The English Physician Enlarged*, an interesting blend of folklore, astrology, and botanical medicine. Both books became extremely popular and are still quoted by herbalists today.

When English settlers arrived in the New World, they exported their knowledge of herbal medicine, which they shared with the Native Americans. Native Americans, in turn, introduced the settlers to many local herbs that were brought back to Europe.

By the 1800s, the Western medical establishment began to turn to chemotherapy—the use of chemical drugs such as mercury, arsenic, and sulphur to cure disease. Herbal medicine, however, continued to be practiced by people who either couldn't afford conventional medical care or who preferred it over modern medical practices. In the United States, the Eclectics, a group of physicians who were prominent until the 1930s, still favored plant medicines, but they were a dying breed. Only homeopathic physicians, who follow the teachings of eighteenth-century physician Samuel Hahnemann, and a handful of other "holistic" practitioners continue to rely primarily on drugs derived from plants or animals.

Today, herbal medicine is still the primary source of healthcare for 80 percent of the world's population. As Westerners become more global in outlook, there is renewed interest in the traditional healing practices of other nations.

NICHOLAS CULPEPER: A MAN FOR ALL SEASONS

Nicholas Culpeper (1616–1654) earned the wrath of the English medical establishment after the publication of his two works, *The English Physician,* a "people's herbal" and an English translation of the *Latin Pharmacopeia,* which up until then, was not widely available to the public. A medical school dropout, Culpeper opened an apothecary in 1640 where he dispensed low-cost botanical medicines. Culpeper's iconoclastic approach to medicine—and his willingness to share information with the people—made him very popular with the public, but he was despised by the medical profession.

Critics were quick to dismiss Culpeper as a quack because his herbal incorporated astrology with healing. Despite the bizarre astrological references, Culpeper's knowledge of plant medicines and their uses showed a great deal of sophistication for his time. Culpeper fought on the Parliamentary side during the English Civil War and suffered a chest wound, which undoubtedly contributed to his early death. Culpeper is still regarded as a folk hero in England.

In 1927, Mrs. C. F. Leyel, founder of the Society of Herbalists in London, opened a shop called Culpepers in memory of the great herbalist. Her aim was "to revive the taste for wholesome natural medicines, pure cosmetics, and the use of herbs in cooking to form a counterattraction to the modern craze for strong synthetic scents." Today, Culpeper's is probably the best-known herbal shop in the world. Nearly four centuries later, Culpeper's herbal is still selling briskly.

CHAPTER 2

The "Hot Hundred"

Literally thousands of herbs are used throughout the world, far too many to list in a single book. In this chapter, I have narrowed the list down to the "Hot Hundred," the herbs that I feel have the potential to make the most significant contribution to our lives. Listed in alphabetical order, many of these herbs offer treatments and remedies for the ailments that most concern us today. You may already be familiar with some of these herbs—some may even be in your kitchen cabinet. Others may seem a bit strange at first, but as you learn more about them, they will seem no more exotic than the rows and rows of synthetic chemical remedies found in any modern pharmacy. All of these herbs can be found in herb shops or health food stores in easy-to-use forms. After reading this chapter, you will see how simple it can be to incorporate herbs into your lifestyle.

HOW TO USE THE "HOT HUNDRED"

For each of the herbs listed in the "Hot Hundred," I have included specific instructions on its appropriate use. However, the capsule or tablet size, or strength of a particular herbal product, may vary from manufacturer to manufacturer. Therefore, if you buy a packaged herb that recommends a different dose, follow the directions on the label. Unless otherwise specified, herbal extracts and powders can be mixed in juice, water, or made into a tea. (For information on how to make an herbal tea, see page 24). They can be sweetened with honey or sugar according to taste. Warm beverages are the drink of choice for colds, coughs, menstrual cramps, and at bedtime.

Under the heading of "Personal Advice" I have listed any personal experience I may have had with a particular herb, or other pertinent anecdotal material.

CAUTION

Some of the "Hot Hundred" herbs are reputed to have anticancer activity and may even be used to treat some forms of cancer in the United States and abroad. Anyone who is receiving treatment for cancer should not discontinue conventional treatment or use any herbs in conjunction with their treatment unless they are under the direction of a qualified oncologist. Parents should not give herbs to children without first checking with their pediatricians. Pregnant women should not take any herbs without asking their obstetricians.

ALFALFA

(Medicago sativa)

FACTS

First discovered by the Arabs, who dubbed this valuable plant the "father of all foods," the leaves of the alfalfa plant are rich in minerals and nutrients, including calcium, magnesium, potassium, and beta carotene (useful against both heart disease and cancer). English herbalist John Gerard (1597) recommended alfalfa for upset stomachs. Noted biologist and author Frank Bouer discovered that the leaves of this remarkable legume contained eight essential amino acids. Alfalfa is a good laxative and a natural diuretic. It is often used to treat urinary tract infections. This versatile herb is also a folk remedy for arthritis, and is reputed to be an excellent appetite stimulant and overall tonic. Unfortunately, most westerners regard alfalfa as cattle fodder, and therefore, rarely take advantage of the beneficial properties of this common plant.

POSSIBLE BENEFITS

Good for cystitis or inflammation of the bladder.

Boosts a sluggish appetite.

Provides relief from bloating or water retention.

Excellent source of nutrients.

Relieves constipation.

May reduce swelling and inflammation of rheumatism.

How to Use It

ORALLY

CAPSULES OR TABLETS:
   Take 3 to 6 daily.
DRIED HERB:
   Mix 1 tablespoon with 8 ounces of warm water. Drink
   1 cup home brewed tea daily.
FRESH:
   Toss alfalfa sprouts in salads.

CAUTION

Alfalfa has been known to aggravate lupus and other auto-immune disorders. If you have an autoimmune problem, avoid this herb.

PERSONAL ADVICE

For relief from rheumatoid arthritis, take 9 to 18 alfalfa tablets daily.

ALMOND
(*Prunus amygdalus*)

If you find commercial soap products too drying for your face, check in your local health food store for facial soaps and cleansers derived from almond. The kernel from the almond plant provides us with one of the best face scrubs Mother Nature has to offer. It is also an excellent emollient. A recent study suggests that almond oil may also help prevent heart disease. At the Health Research and Studies Center in Los Altos, California, almond oil was shown to lower serum cholesterol levels in people who consumed it in place of saturated fat. According to this study, almond oil was a more potent cholesterol-reducing agent than olive oil! More studies are needed to determine if almond oil should be part of a heart-healthy lifestyle.

POSSIBLE BENEFITS

Cleansers made from almond help to remove excess oil and dirt from skin.

Almond butter and oil can moisturize and soften skin.

Almond oil shows promise as a potent cholesterol reducer.

How to Use It

EXTERNALLY

ALMOND MEAL:
   A handful of almond meal makes a good face scrub.
OIL:
   Rub almond oil directly into rough areas, such as hands and heels of feet.

ALOE VERA

(*Aloe barbadenis*)

I have perfumed my bed with myrrh, aloes and cinnamon.
PROVERBS 7:17

FACTS

For more than 3,500 years, healers and physicians have touted the benefits of this fragrant desert lily. There are about two hundred species of this amazing plant, but the aloe vera, meaning "true aloe" in Latin, is considered the most effective healer. The leaf of aloe contains the special "gel" or emollient that is used externally in cosmetics and skin creams. Aloe gel is regarded as one of nature's best natural moisturizers. The bitter juice, which is extracted from the whole leaf, may be taken internally for digestive disorders. Two thousand years ago, the Greek physician Dioscorides wrote that aloe vera was an effective treatment for everything from constipation to burns to kidney ailments. Queen Cleopatra regarded the gel as a fountain of youth and used it to preserve her skin against the ravages of the Egyptian sun. The Egyptians were also believed to have used the aloe plant in their embalming process. The Bible is full of references to aloe, and it is still widely used in Africa to heal burns and wounds. Aloe vera has been used successfully in the United States to treat radiation burns. A recent study in the *Journal of Dermatological Surgery and Oncology* shows that aloe vera significantly speeded the healing process on patients who underwent facial dermabrasion—the removal of the top layers of skin to remove scars.

POSSIBLE BENEFITS

Soothes and promotes healing of sunburn and other kinds of minor burns.

Useful for bug bites and mild skin irritations.

Helps keep skin soft and supple.

Taken internally, aloe is an effective laxative and promotes general healing.

How to Use It

ORALLY

CAPSULES:
Take 1 capsule up to 3 times daily.
JUICE OR GEL:
Take 1 tablespoon up to 3 times daily.

EXTERNALLY

GEL:
Aloe vera gel may be used liberally as needed.

CAUTION

Do not take aloe internally during pregnancy. Aloe should not be used internally by children or the elderly.

PERSONAL ADVICE

There are many so-called aloe vera preparations on the market that contain very little of this precious herb. Some contain only a minute quantity of aloe; others contain "aloe extract," or "reconstituted aloe vera," watered-down versions that are not as beneficial as bona fide aloe gel. A true aloe product should list aloe vera as a primary ingredient—as the first or second ingredient listed on the label—or state that it is 97 to 99 percent pure aloe vera.

ANGELICA

(Angelica archangelica)

FACTS

This herb is named after Archangel Raphael, who according to a tenth-century French legend, revealed the secrets of this herb to a monk for use during a plague epidemic. Angelica is one of nature's most versatile herbs. It is recommended by herbalists for indigestion and stomach upsets. It is also an excellent expectorant. The famous English herbalist Culpeper noted that it "helpeth the pleurisy, as also all other diseases of the lungs and breast." Angelica has a warming effect on the body. It promotes circulation of blood to the extremities and has traditionally been given to people suffering from cold hands and feet due to anemia. Women use angelica to alleviate painful menstrual cramps. Applied externally, it may provide relief from pain and swelling caused by rheumatism. It is also useful for skin lice; it will relieve itching while getting rid of the troublesome pests.

POSSIBLE BENEFITS

Relieves buildup of phlegm due to asthma and bronchitis.

Antispasmodic action relieves menstrual cramps.

Good remedy for skin lice.

Reduces discomfort caused by rheumatism.

Good for people who get cold easily.

How to Use It

ORALLY

EXTRACT:
Mix 10 to 30 drops of extract in liquid, 3 times daily.

EXTERNALLY

EXTRACT:
Rub liquid directly on affected areas.

CAUTION

Do not use during pregnancy. Large doses can affect blood pressure, heart action, and respiration. To avoid these problems, do not exceed recommended dose.

ANISE

(Pimpinella anisum)

FACTS

Since the ancient Egyptians, the sweet-tasting anise seed has been used both as a spice and as a popular remedy. A tea brewed from the crushed seed can relieve digestive disorders and cramps. It also helps loosen phlegm and is useful against coughs and colds. Herbalists recommend anise to soothe colicky infants. Since the Middle Ages, anise tea has been sipped by nursing mothers to increase milk production. This old wive's tale appears to be based on fact: A recent study done at Auburn University shows that cows sprayed with anise oil produced more milk than cows sprayed with other fragrances.

POSSIBLE BENEFITS

Helps expel gas.

Promotes digestion.

Relieves nausea and abdominal pain.

Soothes coughs and colds, helps clear congestion.

Stimulates milk production in nursing mothers.

How to Use It

ORALLY

SEEDS:
Crush seeds into powder. Put 1 teaspoon into 1 cup boiling water. Drink up to 3 times daily.

APPLE

(Pyrus malus)

FACTS

The adage "An apple a day will keep the doctor away" may very well be true. In the second century, Galen, the famous court physician to the emperors and the gladiators, prescribed apple wine as a cure-all for nearly every ailment. While I wouldn't go quite that far in endorsing this fruit (or its wine), I believe that an apple can be an important part of your daily diet. For one thing, it's good for digestion. Depending on how it's used, it can relieve both constipation and diarrhea. Apples are also rich in soluble fiber, a substance that helps regulate blood sugar, preventing a sudden increase or drop in serum sugar levels. Pectin, a type of soluble fiber found in apples, has received much attention lately because of its ability to lower blood cholesterol levels, thus reducing the risk of heart disease. Apples also are a traditional remedy for rheumatism.

POSSIBLE BENEFITS

Helps regulate normal bowel function.

Helps prevent both diarrhea and constipation.

Reduces cholesterol and normalizes blood sugar.

Traditional remedy for joint pain and stiffness due to rheumatism.

How to Use It

ORALLY

For diarrhea, eat a grated, peeled apple. Dried apple peels simmered in warm water help regulate digestion. For maximum benefit, eat 1 to 2 medium-sized apples every day.

ARNICA

(*Arnica montana*)

FACTS

The flower and root of this plant have been used by natural healers as a pain reliever, expectorant, and stimulant. Modern herbalists, however, believe that arnica is very strong medicine, and should not be taken internally unless it is under the supervision of a homeopathic physician. An overdose can be fatal. Rubbed on the skin, however, arnica is wonderful for healing wounds, bruises, or other skin irritations. Commercially prepared liniments may also be used for muscle soreness or arthritis.

POSSIBLE BENEFITS

Soothes and heals skin wounds and irritations.

Relieves pain due to muscle spasm or joint inflammation.

Used internally, it's good for coughs.

How to Use It

EXTERNALLY

There are several commercially prepared salves or ointments that are safe to use externally as needed. An ointment that is too strong will cause further irritation. Therefore, I do not recommend that people prepare their own salves.

CAUTIONS

Never apply arnica on broken skin. If further irritation develops, discontinue use. *Never take arnica internally unless it is under the supervision of a physician.*

ARTICHOKE

(Cynara scolymus)

FACTS

The flower or head of the artichoke—commonly known as the heart—is reputed to be an aphrodisiac, although this claim has never been scientifically proven. Even if this popular vegetable is not good for affairs of the heart, it is certainly good for the heart itself. Through the years, various studies worldwide have shown that people's blood cholesterol levels dropped after eating artichoke. In fact, an anticholesterol drug called cynara is derived from this herb. In 1940, a study in Japan showed that artichoke not only reduced cholesterol but it also increased bile production by the liver and worked as a good diuretic.

POSSIBLE BENEFITS

Relieves excess water weight.

Promotes heart health by reducing cholesterol.

Enhances liver function.

May enhance sexual desire.

How to Use It

ORALLY

To make a delicious, heart-healthy treat, rub the leaves with olive oil and tuck a few slices of garlic in the leaves. Steam for 30 to 40 minutes. Remember that the benefits of this vegetable will be lost if you douse it in melted butter, which is high in saturated fat, or in margarine, which is high in calories.

ASPARAGUS
(Asparagus officinalis)

FACTS

Asparagus is a highly regarded herb worldwide. Chinese pharmacists save the best roots of the asparagus plant for their families and friends in the belief that it will increase feelings of compassion and love. In India, this herb is used to promote fertility, reduce menstrual cramping, and increase milk production in nursing mothers. In the Western world, it has been touted as an aphrodisiac. These customs and beliefs are not mere superstition: Asparagus root contains compounds called steroidal glycosides that directly affect hormone production and may very well influence emotions. An excellent diuretic, asparagus is also very nutritious. It is high in folic acid, which is essential for the production of new red blood cells. Many herbal healers recommend asparagus root for rheumatism, due to the antiinflammatory action of the steroidal glycosides. Powdered seed from the asparagus plant is good for calming an upset stomach.

POSSIBLE BENEFITS

Stimulates hormone production.

Helps rid the body of excess water and salt.

Helps prevent anemia due to folic acid deficiency.

Soothes pain and swelling of joints due to rheumatism or arthritis.

How to Use It

ORALLY

Eat the young shoots and seeds. The seed is available in powder form. Take 1 teaspoon powder daily in juice.

CAUTION

Do not use if your kidneys are inflamed, because it increases the rate of urinary production.

ASTRAGALUS

(Astragalus membranaceous)

FACTS

Grown in China, Oriental herbalists have used astragalus for centuries for a wide variety of ailments, including diabetes, heart disease, and high blood pressure. Westerners, however, are just beginning to discover its many benefits. Recent studies in leading Chinese medical journals suggest that astragalus may help activate the immune system, thus enhancing the body's natural ability to fight disease. Astragalus may also prevent the spread of malignant cancer cells to healthy tissue. Dr. G. Mavligit at the University of Texas in Houston found that an extract from this plant helped restore normal immune function in cancer patients with impaired immunity. In fact, some herbalists routinely give astragalus to people undergoing chemotherapy and radiation. More research is underway to explore the full medical potential of this ancient cure-all.

POSSIBLE BENEFITS

Promotes resistance against disease.

Mild stimulant.

May reduce blood pressure by helping to rid the body of excess water weight.

Appears to help restore normal immune function for cancer patients.

How to Use It

ORALLY

CAPSULES:
Take 1 to 3 (400 mg) capsules daily.

CAUTION

If you are undergoing chemotherapy, do not take astragalus or any other medication without first consulting a doctor who is familiar with this herb.

THE HEART HERB

In 1775, English physician William Withering diagnosed a patient with congestive heart failure as hopeless and sent him home to die. A short time later, he learned that a local folk healer had cured his patient using a bunch of mysterious herbs. Amazed by the man's miraculous recovery, Withering investigated the herbs used by the healer and isolated foxglove (*Digitalis purpurea*) as the main ingredient. After performing several experiments, Withering discovered that this purple-flowered plant was a potent cardiotonic, that is, it improved the heart's pumping action, helping to rid the body of the excess fluid causing the congestion. Withering also learned that in the wrong dose, foxglove could be lethal, triggering a fatal arrhythmia or irregularity in the heartbeat. For the next decade, Withering conducted numerous experiments to determine the precise amount of this drug needed to treat heart failure. He published his results in 1785, informing other physicians of this amazing new cure. Today, digitalis, the drug derived from foxglove, is a highly regarded treatment for heart failure. Due to its unpredictable effect on the heart, the herb should never be consumed without a doctor's supervision.

BASIL
(*Ocimum basilicum*)

FACTS

The word *basil* is derived from the Greek word *king,* suggesting that the ancient healers held this aromatic plant in high regard. Today we think of basil as something that you either sprinkle over tomato sauce or pound into a pesto. Fresh basil is delicious to eat, but the herb is also an effective remedy for a variety of digestive disorders, including stomach cramps, vomiting, and constipation.

POSSIBLE BENEFITS

Reduces stomach cramps and nausea.

Relieves gas.

Promotes normal bowel function.

Aids digestion

How to Use It

ORALLY

DRIED HERB:
Mix 1 teaspoon of dried herbs in ½ cup water. Strain. Drink 1 to 2 cups as needed daily.

BAYBERRY BARK
(*Myrica certifera*)

FACTS

One of the most versatile herbs, this native American plant is highly regarded by herbal practitioners. Nineteenth-century physicians used to prescribe a hot tea made from the powdered bark of the bayberry at the first sign of a cold, cough, or flu. The tea is an excellent expectorant. It also promotes perspiration, helping you literally to sweat out a cold, and is good for circulation. In large doses, bayberry can induce vomiting and was at one time used to treat cases of poisoning. Bayberry makes an excellent mouthwash that is particularly soothing for sore or sensitive gums. Rubbed on the skin, bayberry can be used to reduce the swelling or discomfort caused by varicose veins. It is also one of the oldest remedies for hemorrhoids.

POSSIBLE BENEFITS

Helps clear congestion in chest due to cold.

Has a mild stimulating effect.

Good astringent.

Soothes inflamed varicose veins.

How to Use It

ORALLY

CAPSULES:
   Take 1 capsule up to 3 times daily as needed.
EXTRACT:
   Mix 10 to 20 drops in juice or water.
MOUTHWASH:
   Gargle with liquid mixture made of extract or powder as needed.
POWDER:
   Mix ½ to 1 teaspoon in 1 cup warm water.

EXTERNALLY

Rub liquid mixture on varicose veins or hemorrhoids as needed.

BILBERRY

(Vaccinium myrtillus)

FACTS

Bilberry is a well-known folk remedy for poor vision, especially for people who suffer from "night blindness," that is, they have difficulty seeing in the dark. In fact, bilberry jam was given to Royal Air Force pilots who flew nighttime missions during World War II. Bilberry works by accelerating the regeneration of retinol purple—commonly known as visual purple—a substance that is required for good eyesight. European medical journals are filled with studies confirming bilberry's positive effect on vision. Unfortunately, this herb has not received the attention it deserves in the American medical community.

POSSIBLE BENEFITS

Helps preserve eyesight and prevent eye damage.

Particularly useful for people who suffer from eyestrain or poor night vision.

Good for people who must drive at night

Helpful for nearsightedness (myopia).

How to Use It

ORALLY

CAPSULES:
  Take 1 capsule up to 3 times daily.
EXTRACT:
  Mix 15 to 40 drops in water or juice, and drink 3
  times daily.

CAUTION

Although the commercially prepared extract is safe, the leaves can be poisonous if consumed over a long period of time. Therefore, safety dictates that you not exceed the recommended dosage.

BLACK COHOSH

(Cimicifuga racemosa)

FACTS

Native Americans used this herb to reduce the pain and inflammation of rheumatism and to treat an assortment of "female complaints." Black cohosh is a traditional remedy to induce menstruation, relieve menstrual cramps, and facilitate labor and delivery. Combined with skullcap, wood betony, passionflower, and valerian, black cohosh works as a mild tranquilizer. Herbalists have also used black cohosh to treat persistent coughs in cases of asthma, bronchitis, and whooping cough.

POSSIBLE BENEFITS

Relieves swelling and soreness typical of rheumatism.

Helps you to relax.

Relieves muscle spasm.

Reduces pain associated with neuralgia.

Helps to relax bronchial tubes and quells the urge to cough.

Promotes labor and eases delivery.

How to Use It

ORALLY

CAPSULES:
   Take 1 capsule up to 3 times daily.
EXTRACT:
   Mix 10 to 30 drops of extract in liquid daily.

CAUTION

Large doses can cause symptoms of poisoning. Do not use during pregnancy until labor and only under the supervision of a doctor.

BLACK WALNUT

(Juglans nigra)

FACTS

The fruit, leaves, and bark of this tree offer many benefits. Taken internally, black walnut helps relieve constipation and is also useful against fungal and parasitic infections. It may also help eliminate warts, which are troublesome growths caused by viruses. Rubbed on the skin, black walnut extract is reputed to be beneficial for eczema, herpes, psoriasis, and skin parasites.

POSSIBLE BENEFITS

Fights against fungal infection.

Antiseptic properties help fight bacterial infection.

Antiparasitic.

Helps promote bowel regularity.

How to Use It

ORALLY

EXTRACT:
Mix 10 to 20 drops in water or juice daily.

EXTERNALLY

Rub extract on skin 2 times daily.

BLESSED THISTLE
(*Cnicus benedictus*)

FACTS

This herb is one of the oldest folk remedies for the treatment of amenorrhea, which is absence of the menstrual cycle after the onset of menstruation. Blessed thistle stimulates the production of bile by the liver and is often used by folk healers to treat liver disorders. This herb is also reputed to perk up a sluggish appetite, improve circulation, and stimulate memory. Herbalists use blessed thistle to resolve blood clots and to stop bleeding. For menstruation problems, blessed thistle is usually taken in combination with other herbs such as ginger, cramp bark, and blue cohosh root. This herb is often included in commercial herbal preparations designed specifically for women.

POSSIBLE BENEFITS

Helps regulate menstrual cycle.

Used in treating liver problems.

Improves the appetite.

Lowers fevers.

Helps to stop bleeding.

How to Use It

ORALLY

CAPSULES:
  Take 1 up to 3 times daily.
EXTRACT:
  Mix 10 to 20 drops in liquid daily.

CAUTION

Do not use during pregnancy.

BONESET

(Eupatorium perfoliatum)

FACTS

Native Americans introduced the settlers to this New World herb. Its name reflects its use during a particularly harsh strain of flu called "break bone fever." Come cold and flu season, boneset can be invaluable in relieving coughs and upper respiratory congestion, helping to loosen up phlegm, and clearing nasal passages. It also can be used to help reduce a fever. This versatile herb has a calming effect on the body and can relieve constipation.

POSSIBLE BENEFITS

Brings down a fever.

Relieves flu symptoms.

Has a calming effect on the body.

Taken in a warm drink, it is an excellent expectorant.

Taken in a cold drink, it is a mild laxative.

How to Use It

ORALLY

EXTRACT:
Mix 10 to 40 drops in liquid daily.

BUCHU
(Barosma betulina)

FACTS

Almost four hundred years ago, the Hottentots, a native tribe of South Africa, recognized the many healing properties of this aromatic plant. Combined with the "Hot Hundred Herb" uva ursi, buchu is best known as a remedy for urinary disorders including cystitis and prostate-related problems. It also helps reduce bloating and excess water weight and promotes perspiration.

POSSIBLE BENEFITS

Useful for urinary tract infections.

Good diuretic.

Has a stimulating effect on the body.

How to Use It

ORALLY

CAPSULES:
   Take 1 up to 3 times daily.
EXTRACT:
   Mix 10 to 30 drops in juice or water.

CAUTION

Do not use for kidney infections or if you have any kidney problems, since buchu can be irritating to the kidneys. Kidney infections need prompt medical attention. If you have pain during urination, or blood in the urine, call your doctor immediately.

BURDOCK
(*Arctium lappa*)

FACTS

Natural healers revere this herb as nature's best "blood purifier," that is, they believe that it rids the body of dangerous toxins. Ancient herbalists used burdock to treat snake bites. Nicholas Culpeper, the famous seventeenth-century herbalist, wrote that it "helpeth those that are bit by a mad dog." Today, many herbalists still recommend this herb for its diuretic action: It increases the flow of urine and promotes sweating. It is also reputed to be helpful for the soreness and swelling caused by arthritis, rheumatism, sciatica, and lumbago. Used externally, it is considered a major natural treatment for skin problems such as eczema, psoriasis, and even canker sores. Burdock is also soothing for hemorrhoids.

POSSIBLE BENEFITS

Helps rid body of excess water weight.

Soothes pain caused by arthritis, rheumatism, and backache.

Relieves skin irritation.

How to Use It

ORALLY

CAPSULES:
Take 1 to 3 daily.
EXTRACT:
Mix 10 to 25 drops of extract in liquid daily.

EXTERNALLY

Apply locally to inflamed area as needed.

BUTCHER'S BROOM

(Ruscus acluteatus)

FACTS

In Europe, practitioners of folk medicine have relied on this herb for centuries to relieve excess water retention and constipation. Today, it is extremely popular among European women to treat the discomfort and pain caused by poor circulation in the legs—that heavy leg feeling, also known as restless leg syndrome. French scientists discovered that this plant contains steroidal-type compounds that can constrict veins and reduce inflammation. Butcher's broom has also been used to soothe the swelling and pain of arthritis and rheumatism. Taken orally or made into an ointment, it is excellent for the treatment of hemorrhoids.

POSSIBLE BENEFITS

Improves circulation in hands and feet.

Helps reduce edema in legs or feet.

Antiinflammatory action can reduce swelling caused by arthritis and rheumatism.

Reduces pain caused by hemorrhoids.

How to Use It

ORALLY

CAPSULES:
   Take 1 up to 3 times daily.
EXTRACT:
   Mix 10 to 20 drops in liquid daily.

EXTERNALLY

OINTMENT:
  Apply small amounts to hemorrhoids until inflammation is cleared.

PERSONAL ADVICE

This is a particularly good herb for people who are on their feet most of the day—salespersons, teachers, and doctors—and as a result, experience swelling at night.

CALENDULA
(*Calendula officinalis*)

FACTS

Calendula is an essential oil that can be used for many purposes. Used externally, this herb can soothe burns and promote healing of wounds. Applied directly to the ear, calendula oil can reduce the pain and discomfort of an earache. Taken orally, it can help break a fever, quiet an angry ulcer, and relieve menstrual cramps. It can also provide relief from eruptive skin diseases, such as shingles (herpes zoster), which is caused by a virus much like the chicken pox virus.

POSSIBLE BENEFITS

Relieves pain and promotes healing of burns and skin wounds.

Reduces fever.

Quells pain from ulcer irritation.

Reduces menstrual cramps.

How to Use It

ORALLY

DRIED HERB:
   Make tea from 1 heaping tablespoon of dried herb.
   Drink 1 cup daily.
EXTRACT:
   Mix 10 to 30 drops in liquid daily.

EXTERNALLY

Apply oil or commercial preparation directly to affected area daily. Put on cotton swab and place in ear for earache.

CAUTION

Do not use during pregnancy.

CAPSICUM OR CAYENNE
(*Capsicum frutescens*)

FACTS

Contrary to popular belief, hot, spicy food may actually be good for your health, that is, if it contains liberal amounts of cayenne, also known as capsicum. Cayenne is used as an overall digestive aid: It stimulates the production of gastric juices, improves metabolism, and even helps relieve gas. Cayenne is also very nutritious. Peppers in general contain more vitamin C than oranges, as well as iron, calcium, phosphorous, and B-complex vitamins. A meal rich in cayenne will have a mildly stimulating effect on the body. According to Dr. Irwin Ziment of the UCLA School of Medicine, the hot, stinging sensation that follows biting into a chile pepper triggers the release of endorphins by the brain, chemicals that relieve pain and can cause a mild euphoria.

Cayenne tea is excellent for a cold and chills. Cayenne also appears to have a beneficial effect on blood fats. According to a 1987 study published in the *Journal of Bioscience*, rats fed a diet high in cayenne experienced a significant reduction in blood triglycerides and low-density lipoproteins (LDL), or "bad" cholesterol. Capsaicin, a compound found in cayenne that gives the spice its "kick," is an antiinflammatory. Recently, cayenne has been used successfully to treat patients with cluster headaches, a particularly painful type of headache. Used externally, cayenne liniment can soothe the stiffness and pain of rheumatism and arthritis.

POSSIBLE BENEFITS

Soothes indigestion.

Reduces discomfort caused by the common cold.

Stimulates the appetite.

Reduces inflammation.

Mild stimulant or tonic.

How to Use It

ORALLY

CAPSULES:
Take 1 to 3 daily.
TEA:
A cup of tea can be taken for stomach cramps or a cold daily. Prepared teas are available, or make it from dried herb.

EXTERNALLY

LINIMENT:
Rub on affected areas.

CAUTION

Cayenne can be irritating to hemorrhoids. It should not be used by people with gastrointestinal problems. Never apply cayenne ointment to broken skin. Prolonged application can cause skin irritation. If taking internally, do not exceed recommended dose. High dosages taken internally can cause gastroenteritis and kidney damage.

CARAWAY
(*Carum carvi*)

FACTS

The seeds from this plant, which are often used in baked goods, are known for their mildly spicy, aromatic flavor. Caraway is soothing for gas and other stomach disorders. It can also increase the appetite. Brewed into a tea, the warm fluid is excellent for coughs and colds. For centuries, midwives have used caraway to stimulate the production of breast milk in nursing mothers and to ease colic in infants.

POSSIBLE BENEFITS

Excellent digestive aid.

Helps expel gas.

Reduces nausea.

Improves the appetite.

Works as an effective expectorant for coughs due to colds.

Increases breast milk in nursing mothers.

How to Use It

ORALLY

EXTRACT:
   Mix 3 to 4 drops in liquid, 3 to 4 times daily.
   For colic, mix 1 to 2 drops in infant formula for 2
   feedings. (Check with your pediatrician before giving
   this or any other herb to your baby or child.)
SEEDS:
   Chew the seeds 3 to 4 times daily.

CAUTION

Never give seeds to infants or young children—stick to the extract.

THE SPICE OF LIFE

Some well-known herbs have spicy pasts. Caraway seeds were once used in love potions. Coriander, a popular ingredient in salsa, was once a highly regarded aphrodisiac. Even the common onion was at one time prescribed by herbalists to restore sexual potency.

CARROT

(*Daucus carota*)

FACTS

Bugs Bunny was right! Carrots are rich in carotene, a plant form of vitamin A that is believed to help prevent certain types of cancer. Numerous studies worldwide, including some sponsored by the National Cancer Institute, confirm that people who eat diets high in carrots and other foods rich in carotene are less likely to develop certain forms of cancer than those who don't. In fact, studies show that even people who are exposed to specific carcinogens such as tobacco and ultraviolet light could reduce their risk of cancer by eating more carotene.

The RDA (recommended daily allowance) for carotene is 5,000 IU, but cancer researchers suggest that in order to dramatically decrease your cancer risk, you should consume about 12,500 IU a day. (This isn't too difficult considering that one grated, raw carrot daily provides about 13,500 units of carotene.) Carotene is also excellent for the eyes. Carotene permits the formation of visual purple in the eyes, which helps counteract night blindness and weak vision. Three large raw carrots a day may also lower blood cholesterol levels, thus reducing your risk of developing coronary artery disease, the leading cause of heart attack. Carrots are also a good treatment for diarrhea and can relieve gas and heartburn.

POSSIBLE BENEFITS

Promotes eye health.

Helps prevent cancer.

Lowers cholesterol.

Soothes indigestion.

Can help relieve diarrhea.

How to Use It

ORALLY

JUICE:
   Drink 1 to 2 cups daily of homemade (if you have an automatic juicer) or commercially prepared fresh product.
SOUP:
   Boil 1 pound grated carrots and chopped leaves in ¾ cup water until very thick. Strain.

PERSONAL ADVICE

When it comes to carrots, the fresher the product the better. From the minute the carrot is picked, the carotene begins to lose its potency. Try to buy loose carrots from the greengrocer and avoid the stuff that's sold in plastic bags. Use them as quickly as possible.

CASCARA SAGRADA OR BUCKTHORN
(*Rhamnus purshiana*)

FACTS

Cascara, also called buckthorn, works by stimulating the lining of the upper intestines to promote normal bowel function. It is one of nature's milder laxatives and is effective against chronic constipation.

POSSIBLE BENEFITS

Relieves constipation overnight.

How to Use It

ORALLY

CAPSULES OR TABLETS:
Take 1 to 3 daily.

CAUTION

Excessive dose can cause cramps and diarrhea.

PERSONAL ADVICE

In my many years as pharmacist, I have found that the bark from the California buckthorn (cascara sagrada) is still the most effective laxative known. It has also been used for gallstones and liver ailments.

CATNIP
(*Nepeta cataria*)

FACTS

This herb is well known for its ability to drive felines into a frenzy, but it actually has the opposite effect on humans. Catnip is a mild sedative that is useful for cramps and upset stomach. In Europe, this herb is a popular remedy for bronchitis and diarrhea. Catnip promotes sweating and has a warming effect on the body.

POSSIBLE BENEFITS

Helps you relax.

Eases indigestion and gas.

May help relieve bronchitis.

Helps control diarrhea.

How to Use It

ORALLY

CAPSULES:
  Take 1 to 3 daily.
EXTRACT:
  Mix ½ to 1 teaspoon in ½ cup warm water and drink as a tea.

CELERY

(Apium graveolens)

FACTS

Although you may think of celery as nothing more than something crunchy to chop into a salad, the root, leaves, and seeds of this plant offer many health benefits. Celery juice and extract of celery seed are excellent diuretics that promote the flow of urine through the kidneys. Celery has a calming effect on the digestive system, relieving gas and indigestion. It is also reputed to be helpful against rheumatism and gout. Drinking celery juice is a popular folk remedy to promote the onset of menstruation.

POSSIBLE BENEFITS

Natural diuretic.

Good for digestion system and enhances appetite.

May relieve symptoms of rheumatism and gout.

Celery juice and oil induces menstruation.

How to Use It

ORALLY

JUICE:
   Take 1 tablespoon of juice 2 to 3 times daily.
OIL:
   Mix 6 to 8 drops of celery oil in water, and drink twice daily.

CAUTION

Celery juice and oil should not be used during pregnancy.

CHAMOMILE OR CAMOMILE
(*Matricaria chamomilla*)

FACTS

Back in the days when women often came down with a mysterious malady called "the vapors," a cup of chamomile tea was often prescribed to relieve female anxiety. Known for its calming effect on smooth muscle tissue, chamomile is still a popular remedy for nervous stomach, menstrual cramps, and other common problems often related to stress. Since 1600, Europeans have used chamomile as a cure for insomnia, neuralgia, back pain, and rheumatism. They were not the first to discover this herb; the ancient Egyptians included chamomile in their arsenal of herbal cures. Used externally, it is also good for skin inflammations and hemorrhoids. Used as a mouthwash, it can relieve the pain of toothache. Chamomile is put in shampoos to enhance golden highlights of blond hair. A cup of chamomile tea is the perfect nightcap!

POSSIBLE BENEFITS

Good for the digestion.

Has a relaxing effect on the body.

Traditional treatment for rheumatism.

Relieves back pain.

Soothes skin irritations.

Good for sunburn.

How to Use It

ORALLY

CAPSULES:
   Take 1 up to 3 times daily.
EXTRACT:
   Mix 10 to 20 drops in water up to 3 times daily.
TEA:
   Drink 1 cup daily.

EXTERNALLY

Rub extract on skin irritations as needed. Put in bath water to relieve hemorrhoids.

CAUTION

Chamomile is a member of the daisy family, and anyone who is allergic to other members of the daisy family, including ragweed, should steer clear of this herb. If you are unsure, consult your doctor or allergist.

PERSONAL ADVICE

I drink a cup nightly as a sleep aid. In restaurants, chamomile tea is usually available instead of regular tea, which contains caffeine.

CHAPARRAL
(*Larrea tridentata*)

FACTS

The American pioneers learned about this versatile herb from Native Americans. Chaparral contains a powerful antioxidant, nordihydroguaiaretic acid (NDGA). Antioxidants inhibit the formation of dangerous substances in the body called free radicals, which disrupt normal cell function. Free radicals combine at random with components of healthy cells and interfere with normal cell growth. Free radicals are believed to be responsible for certain types of cancerous tumors and premature aging. Antioxidants prevent free radicals from doing their damage, thus helping to slow the growth of tumors and perhaps even retard the aging process. A biochemist in Louisville, Kentucky, who tested the effects of NDGA on female mosquitoes, reported that he was able to double their average life span from 29 days to 45 days. This herb also helps the body ward off infection, fights parasites, and is useful for urinary tract infections and diarrhea. An antiinflammatory, chaparral also relieves pain and swelling caused by arthritis and rheumatism. Externally, it can be applied directly on wounds and injuries.

POSSIBLE BENEFITS

Helps the body fight infection.

Helps prevent parasitic infection.

Rids the body of excess water weight.

Prevents the growth of certain cancerous tumors.

Reduces inflammation.

Helps stop diarrhea.

May help slow down aging process by preventing the formation of free radicals.

How to Use It

ORALLY

CAPSULES:
Take 1 capsule 3 times daily.
EXTRACT:
Mix 10 to 30 drops in liquid 3 times daily.

EXTERNALLY

Apply extract directly on injured skin.

CHIVES

(Allium schoenoprasum)

FACTS

High in vitamin C and iron, these members of the lily family can easily be grown at home in a window box or can be found fresh at most greengrocers or supermarkets. Chives stimulate the appetite and aid in digestion. High in iron, they are useful against anemia. First discovered in China five thousand years ago, chives later became popular in Europe not only for their subtle onion flavor but because of the widespread belief that their grasslike leaves could chase away evil spirits and disease. It was not uncommon to find clusters of chives hanging from ceilings and bedposts.

POSSIBLE BENEFITS

Good for the digestion.

Helps prevent anemia caused by iron deficiency.

How to Use It

ORALLY

Chop up and sprinkle on salads or over food.

PERSONAL ADVICE

In order to receive maximum benefit, chives must be eaten fresh. This is one that you could even grow at home!

CLOVES

(Caryophyllum aromaticus)

FACTS

Cloves are actually the dried buds of the clove tree. Used in China for more than two thousand years, legend has it that cloves are an aphrodisiac. Although there isn't any evidence to back up this claim, we do know that oil of clove is a time-honored remedy for toothache. Clove oil is highly antiseptic. It is also used to stop vomiting.

POSSIBLE BENEFITS

Relieves tooth pain.

Has an antiemetic action that helps control vomiting.

How to Use It

ORALLY

OIL:
   For toothache, rub oil on affected area. For vomiting, mix 2 drops of oil in a cup of water.

COMFREY

(Symphytum officinale)

FACTS

Generations of herbal healers have used comfrey to treat skin wounds without ever knowing why this plant is so effective. We now know that comfrey contains allantoin, a substance that helps stimulate the growth of new cells and is now used in many cosmetic products. Commercially prepared comfrey creams and ointments are useful for all kinds of skin irritations, including chafing and bug bites. External comfrey preparations have also been used to promote healing of damaged tendons or ligaments.

At one time, comfrey was taken internally for ulcers and irritable bowel syndrome. Today, we are more cautious about ingesting comfrey because it contains pyrroliziidine alkaloids, compounds known to cause liver disease if taken over a long period of time. In 1978, the National Cancer Institute reported that rats fed comfrey roots or leaves developed liver cancer. In fact, in the 1980s, two medical journals—*Gastroenterology* in the United States and the *British Medical Journal*—reported two cases of liver damage resulting from the frequent consumption of comfrey-pepsin tablets for gastrointestinal disorders. In Canada, Russian comfrey, which contains high levels of pyrroliziidine, has been banned. Common comfrey, which contains much lower levels of this dangerous substance, is still sold freely.

In the United States, the FDA is investigating pyrroliziidine alkaloid levels in domestic comfrey. Due to its potential cancer hazard, the internal use of comfrey is a controversial subject among herbalists. Some believe that it should never be ingested. Others, however, feel that in low doses it is harmless as compared to other substances. Proponents of comfrey cite a 1987 study reported in *Science* magazine that rated carcinogens based on their potential risk. Noted carcinogen authority Bruce Ames of the University of California estimated that one cup of comfrey tea was about as risky as eating one peanut butter sandwich, which has traces of estragole, a natural carcinogen. In light of the uncertainty over its safety, however, I believe that comfrey should not be taken internally, especially since there are other safer herbs that can be used in its place, such as peppermint, balm, and ginger.

POSSIBLE BENEFITS

Promotes healing of skin wounds.

Soothes skin irritations.

Relieves ulcers.

How to Use It

EXTERNALLY

Use prepared ointment or extract on skin wounds, insect bites, chafing, or other irritations.

PERSONAL ADVICE

Some comfrey salves on the market specifically recommend use by nursing mothers with chafed nipples. However, since comfrey should not be ingested by infants, I would advise against this use.

CRANBERRY

(Vaccinium macrocarpon)

FACTS

Americans eat about 117 million pounds of cranberry sauce each year, most of it during November and December. But don't wait for Thanksgiving—the common cranberry is one of nature's best weapons against cystitis and urinary tract infections. For years, doctors have routinely advised patients to drink cranberry juice to prevent urinary infections. In fact, it is cited as an effective remedy for this problem in the *U.S. Pharmacopeia*, the official listing of drugs in the United States. At one time, scientists believed that cranberry acidified the urine, and in the process, killed invading bacteria that could cause infection. Recently, however, Dr. Anthony Sabota, a scientist at Youngstown State University in Ohio, offered another possible explanation. His studies suggest that cranberry prevents bacteria from sticking to the wall of the bladder, thus flushing the potential troublemakers out of the body before they can do their damage. At this writing, no one knows precisely how cranberry works, but nearly everyone agrees that it does. Unfortunately, commercially prepared cranberry juice beverages are often laden with sugar and high in calories. Capsules of cranberry extract available in health food stores are not only more potent but less caloric.

POSSIBLE BENEFITS

Prevents the spread of bacterial infection in the urinary tract.

How to Use It

ORALLY

CAPSULES:
Take 1 up to 3 times daily.

CAUTION

If you suspect that you have a urinary infection, see your doctor at once. Untreated, it can lead to serious complications.

PERSONAL ADVICE

The cranberry juice cocktails sold in grocery stores are highly sweetened and processed. This is definitely not the kind of juice I advise people to use. Look for unsweetened, unprocessed products in specialty food stores or health food stores. Real cranberry juice is very tart, but it is also very effective. Some health food stores carry a natural, unprocessed cranberry juice–apple juice combination beverage, which is okay to use as long as it contains no added sugar.

DAMIANA

(Turnera aphrodisiaca)

FACTS

As its botanical name suggests, damiana is reputed to be a sexual stimulant and folk cure for impotence. This herb is also put to more mundane uses: Herbalists recommend it as both a laxative and as a general tonic to improve overall body function. Some herbalists believe that it helps relieve anxiety and promotes a feeling of well-being.

POSSIBLE BENEFITS

May enhance sexual performance.

Helps relieve constipation.

May put you in a good mood!

How to Use It

ORALLY

CAPSULES:
    Take 1 up to 3 times daily before meals.
EXTRACT:
    Mix 10 to 30 drops in liquid daily.

DANDELION
(*Taraxacum officinale*)

FACTS

Dandelion is a natural diuretic and digestive aid. Its high mineral content may help prevent iron-deficiency anemia. This herb also reduces high blood pressure, probably due to its diuretic action. Dandelion is rich in potassium, which works with sodium to regulate the body's water balance and normalize heart rhythms. This vital mineral is often flushed from the body by synthetic diuretics. Dandelion enhances liver and gallbladder function and has traditionally been used by herbal healers to treat liver disorders such as jaundice (a condition caused by an excess amount of bile in the blood). Dandelion is rich in lecithin, a substance researchers believe may protect against cirrhosis of the liver.

POSSIBLE BENEFITS

Helps rid body of excess water and salt.

May decrease high blood pressure by ridding the body of excess fluid, thus reducing the amount of fluid the heart must pump to circulate blood.

Good for the digestion.

Protects against liver and gallbladder disorders.

May protect against iron-deficiency anemia.

How to Use It

ORALLY

CAPSULES:
Take 1 up to 3 times daily.
EXTRACT:
Mix 10 to 30 drops in juice or water daily.

PERSONAL ADVICE

A combination of dandelion root, ginseng, and ginger root has worked wonders for people suffering from low blood sugar, along with a sound nutritional diet. A cup of this special blend (using either the extracts or dried herbs) 3 times a day will do the trick.

LOVES ME . . . LOVES ME NOT

Before the days of Ouija boards, the feathery seed balls of the dandelion were used by young maidens to determine if their true loves were really true. A maiden would blow on the dandelion three times. If at least one of the fuzzy seeds remained, it was taken as an omen that her sweetheart was thinking about her.

DEVIL'S CLAW
(*Harpagophytum procumbens*)

FACTS

The root of this herb has been popular in Africa and Europe for more than 250 years, but it is just being discovered in the United States. Devil's claw is primarily used as an antiinflammatory and a painkiller against arthritis and rheumatism. Recent studies done in France and Germany compare its antiinflammatory action to the drugs cortisone and phenylbutazone.

POSSIBLE BENEFITS

Promotes flexibility in the joints, reducing the pain of arthritis and rheumatism.

How to Use It

ORALLY

CAPSULES:
Take 1 up to 3 times daily.

CAUTION

Do not use during pregnancy.

DILL

(*Aniethum graveolens*)

FACTS

Since biblical times, dill has been cultivated for its aromatic seeds. Widely used in cooking, dill is best known as a digestive aid and remedy for a sour, gassy stomach. It is also used to promote milk production in nursing mothers. Chewing dill seeds is an old-time cure for bad breath.

POSSIBLE BENEFITS

Soothes indigestion and upset stomach.

Promotes appetite.

Helps milk production in nursing mothers.

Helps expel gas.

How to Use It

ORALLY

Steep 2 teaspoons dill seeds in 1 cup of water for 10 to 15 minutes. Strain. Take ½ cup 2 to 3 times daily.

DONG QUAI
(*Angelica sinensis*)

FACTS

Dubbed the "female ginseng," dong quai is an all-purpose herb for a wide range of female gynecological complaints. For centuries, Chinese women have used this herb to regulate the menstrual cycle and quell painful menstrual cramps caused by uterine contractions. Modern herbalists use dong quai to eliminate the discomfort of premenstrual syndrome (PMS) and to help women resume normal menstruation after going off "the pill." Dong quai is also reputed to be useful against hot flashes and other symptoms of menopause caused by hormonal changes. Rich in vitamins and minerals including A, B_{12}, and E, this herb may also prevent anemia. Dong quai has also been used to treat insomnia and high blood pressure for both sexes. Both men and women use this herb as a blood tonic. One of the most widely used herbs in the Orient, dong quai duck is a popular Cantonese dish.

POSSIBLE BENEFITS

Overall tonic for female reproductive system.

Restores menstrual regularity.

Reduces PMS.

Relieves symptoms of menopause.

Prevents anemia.

Reduces high blood pressure.

How to Use It

ORALLY

CAPSULES:
Take 1 up to 3 times daily.

CAUTION

Do not use during pregnancy or if you are still menstru-
ating and typically have a heavy flow.

ECHINACEA
(*Echinacea angustifolia*)

FACTS

We owe Native Americans a debt of gratitude for intro-
ducing the settlers to the wonders of this purple cone-
flower plant. Indians of the Great Plains first used this
herb as a remedy for snakebites and other skin wounds.
They also applied the root of this plant directly to the
mouth for toothaches and sore throats. Word of echinacea's healing properties traveled back to Europe where it is
one of the most sought-after herbs and one of the better
researched as well.

There is renewed interest in echinacea today in the
United States because of this herb's positive effect on the
immune system. Many studies have shown that echinacea
prevents the formation of an enzyme called hyaluroni-
dase, which destroys a natural barrier between healthy
tissue and unwanted pathogenic organisms. Thus, echinacea helps the body maintain its line of defense against
unwanted invaders, especially viruses. In 1972, a study

appeared in the *Journal of Medical Chemistry* showing that an echinacea extract inhibited tumor growth in rats. Echinacea has also been used to help restore normal immune function in patients receiving chemotherapy. In 1978, a study in *Planta Medica* showed that a root extract destroyed both herpes and influenza viruses.

Several European studies show that echinacea appears to lessen the severity of colds and flu, and helps speed recovery. Echinacea has also been used successfully to treat candida, an annoying and persistent fungal infection. In fact, patients treated with an antifungal cream and echinacea extract were less likely to suffer a recurrence than those treated solely with the antifungal cream. Other studies show that echinacea has been used successfully to treat psoriasis and eczema.

POSSIBLE BENEFITS

Boosts the immune system.

Promotes healing of skin wounds.

Fights bacterial and viral infections.

Shortens the duration of colds and flu.

How to Use It

ORALLY

CAPSULES:
Take 1 capsule 3 times daily.
EXTRACT:
Mix 15 to 30 drops in liquid every 3 hours.

PERSONAL ADVICE

Many of the active compounds in echinacea can be destroyed during processing. Freeze drying is the most effective way to preserve this herb's healing properties. A fully potent echinacea preparation will create a tingling sensation on the tongue. If yours doesn't, you're missing out on some important compounds.

ELDER

(*Sambuccua canadensis nigra*)

FACTS

For centuries, the berry from the elderberry tree has been a popular Gypsy remedy for colds, influenza, and neuralgia. The hot tea promotes sweating and is soothing for upper respiratory infections. Externally, it has been used to relieve skin inflammations such as eczema. In ancient times, elderberry trees were believed to have special mystical properties and it was considered good luck to plant a tree near your house to protect against disease and evil spirits. There is one planted outside of Westminster Abbey for this purpose. Judas is said to have hung himself from this type of tree. Elderberries are also a good source of vitamins A, B, and C. Cooked berries can be used in pies and jams.

POSSIBLE BENEFITS

Relieves symptoms of coughs and colds.

Applied externally, useful for burns, rashes, and minor skin problems.

THE LEGEND OF THE ELDER

The elder tree was reputed to be the favorite tree of witches, who supposedly resided in its branches. In the Middle Ages, nearly everyone knew that cutting down an elder tree would incur the wrath of the witches who called it home. There were many tales of angry witches taking vengeance on babies whose unwitting parents put them in a cradle of elder wood.

How to Use It

ORALLY

A liquid made of elderberry juice boiled together with crabapple and a little sugar to form a syrup is an old Gypsy remedy for coughs and bronchial infections, but store-bought elderberry tea and honey will also do the trick.

EXTERNALLY

Elderberry ointments may be used to relieve dry skin.

CAUTION

The seeds from the raw elderberry plant are toxic; therefore, don't eat the berry unless it is cooked. Store-bought elderberry preparations (teas, salves) are perfectly safe.

EPHEDRA
(Ephedra sinica)

FACTS

Known as ma huang in China where it is grown in the Inner Mongolia region, this herb has been used for more than four thousand years to treat asthma and upper respiratory infections. Ephedra, which is cultivated in the dry regions of North America, contains two alkaloids—ephedrine and pseudoephedrine—which today are used in many over-the-counter cold and allergy medications. Also called "Mormon tea" and "Squaw tea," American ephedra was discovered by the early pioneers and Mormon settlers, who used it to treat asthma. It is also useful for headaches, fevers, and hayfever.

POSSIBLE BENEFITS

Decongestant can relieve stuffy nose, watery eyes, and other cold and allergy symptoms.

May help relieve headaches.

Long-acting stimulant that can last up to 24 hours.

How to Use It

ORALLY

CAPSULES:
Take 1 up to 3 times daily to relieve symptoms.
COLD REMEDIES:
Ephedra teas and other commercially prepared cold remedies are sold in health food and herb stores.

CAUTION

Do not use this herb if you have high blood pressure, heart disease, diabetes, or thyroid disease unless under the supervision of your doctor. Do not exceed recommended dose. If you are pregnant or nursing, check with your doctor before using any ephedra preparations.

EUCALYPTUS
(*Eucalyptus globulus*)

FACTS

Koala bears eat them, but human beings have relied on the leaves of this plant for a wide range of medicinal purposes. The oil of eucalyptus and its active ingredient, eucalyptol, are frequently found in over-the-counter cough drops and salves. The oil is also commonly used in steam inhalation preparations for colds and flu—a few whiffs is often all it takes to clear a stuffy nose and a foggy head. Rubbed on the skin, eucalyptus oil provides relief against the pain of arthritis and rheumatism. It increases blood flow to the area, thus producing a feeling of warmth. When aged, the oil forms ozone, a form of oxygen that specifically destroys bacteria, fungi, and viruses.

POSSIBLE BENEFITS

Helps relieve upper respiratory distress caused by cold and flu.

Good expectorant.

Good antiseptic.

Can help soothe stiffness and swelling of arthritis and rheumatism.

How to Take It

EXTERNALLY

Put 1 to 5 drops in a vaporizer. Use liniment as needed.

CAUTION

Do not use on broken or irritated skin. Do not use internally.

PERSONAL ADVICE

Presently, a widely advertised commercial rub contains eucalyptus and mint together in an ointment for arthritis and rheumatism.

EVENING PRIMROSE
(Oenothera biennis)

FACTS

Evening primrose is an American herb that was brought to Europe in the seventeenth century. Once called "king's cure-all," this herb has been used for a wide range of problems. Native Americans used it as a painkiller and asthma treatment. The oil from this plant is high in gamma linolenic acid (GLA), an essential polyunsaturated fatty acid that is converted into prostaglandin, hormones necessary for many important body functions.

Studies have shown that evening primrose oil can help lower blood cholesterol. In fact, according to one Canadian study, patients who took 4 grams of Efamol (a brand of evening primrose oil) daily experienced a 31.5 percent decline in cholesterol after three months of treatment. Other studies have shown that evening primrose oil also reduces blood pressure. Evening primrose is often used to treat symptoms of premenstrual syndrome such as irritability, headaches, breast tenderness, and bloating. It is also used to alleviate anxiety and has been given to schizophrenics with good results. This herb is an old-time remedy for infantile eczema or "cradle cap." A 1987 study in the *British Journal of Dermatology* concluded that patients with eczema showed significant improvement after being treated with evening primrose oil and were able to reduce their dependence on steroids.

POSSIBLE BENEFITS

Relieves symptoms of premenstrual syndrome.

Reduces anxiety.

Helps prevent heart disease and stroke by controlling high blood pressure and reducing cholesterol.

Helps maintain healthy skin.

How to Use It

ORALLY

CAPSULES:
Take 250 mg up to 3 times daily. For PMS, use evening primrose oil 2 to 3 days before symptoms usually appear until the onset of menstruation.

EYEBRIGHT

(Euphrasia officinalis)

FACTS

Since the Middle Ages, eyebright has been used as a tonic and an astringent. It is especially useful for eyestrain, eye inflammations, and other eye ailments. It can greatly relieve runny, sore, itchy eyes due to colds or allergies.

POSSIBLE BENEFITS

An eyewash made of eyebright and other herbs can be soothing to irritated and inflamed eyes.

Taken internally, it may help maintain good vision and eye health.

How to Use It

ORALLY

CAPSULES:
Take 1 up to 3 times daily.
EXTRACT:
Mix 15 to 40 drops in liquid every 3 to 4 hours.

EXTERNALLY

EYEWASHES:
Eyewash products containing euphrasia, plus other herbs such as golden seal, bayberry, raspberry leaves, and cayenne pepper, are available commercially. Put eyewash in eyecup and rinse out eye 3 to 4 times daily.

PERSONAL ADVICE

Hayfever sufferers should try taking this herb for "allergic eyes."

FENNEL

(*Foeniculum vulgare*)

FACTS

Fennel is one of those spices in your kitchen cabinet that can be put to many uses. For centuries, this herb has been used to relieve gas and to stimulate appetite. Fennel oil with honey in warm water is an old-time cough remedy that was used long before the arrival of the over-the-counter "ussins." Used externally, the oil is a folk remedy for joint inflammation due to rheumatism and arthritis.

POSSIBLE BENEFITS

Digestive aid that can relieve cramps and gas.

Good expectorant for coughs and colds.

Can improve a sluggish appetite.

Relieves stiff, painful joints.

How to Use It

ORALLY

EXTRACT:
Mix 10 to 20 drops in water. Use warm water and a teaspoon of honey for a soothing drink daily.

EXTERNALLY

The oil can be rubbed on affected parts of the body as needed to alleviate the pain of arthritis and rheumatism.

FENUGREEK

(Trigonella graecum)

FACTS

One of the oldest known medicinal plants, use of fenugreek dates back to the ancient Egyptians and Hippocrates. A popular folk remedy for sore throats and colds, this herb is also reputed to be an aphrodisiac. Fenugreek may also be useful against diabetes. In a study done in India involving insulin-dependent diabetics on low doses of insulin, pulverized seeds of fenugreek were shown to reduce blood sugar and other harmful fats. The authors of the study suggested that diabetics may benefit by adding fenugreek seeds to their diets. Used externally, pulverized fenugreek seeds may help soothe skin irritations and reduce the pain of neuralgia, swollen glands, and tumors.

POSSIBLE BENEFITS

Good expectorant for coughs and colds.

As a gargle, can relieve sore throat.

Useful for skin irritations and other inflammations.

Lowers blood sugar.

How to Use It

ORALLY

CAPSULES:
Take 1 up to 3 times daily.
GARGLE:
Mix 1 tablespoon of pulverized seed in 8 ounces of hot water. Let steep for 10 minutes. Strain. Gargle 3 times daily every 3–4 hours to relieve sore throat.

EXTERNALLY

The seeds can be pulverized and made into a poultice that can be applied against painful areas of the body. Mix enough pulverized seeds in 8 ounces of warm water to make a thick paste. Apply directly to the affected areas daily.

FEVERFEW

(Chrysanthemum parthenium)

FACTS

Legend has it that this herb saved the life of someone who had the misfortune of falling off the Parthenon, the famous temple in ancient Greece. Since that time, herbalists have used feverfew for a wide variety of problems. As its name suggests, it was used to help bring down a fever. The Greek herbalist Dioscorides is believed to have used this herb to treat arthritis. In 1649, Culpeper recommended it for women as a "general strengthener of their wombs," and also noted that "it is very effectual for all pains in the head." In 1772, John Hill, another famous herbalist, wrote that "in the worst headache, this herb exceeds whatever else is known."

Feverfew was all but forgotten until 1978 when British newspapers told of a woman who had cured her migraines with feverfew leaves. The articles caught the attention of serious medical researchers who decided to further examine this phenomenon. In 1985, the well-respected British medical journal *Lancet* reported that extracts of feverfew inhibited the release of two inflammatory substances— serotonin from platelets and prostaglandin from white blood cells—both thought to contribute to the onset of migraine attacks and perhaps even to play a role in rheumatoid arthritis. In 1988, *Lancet* also reported that a carefully designed study proved what herbalists have known for centuries: Feverfew can help prevent migraine headaches or lessen their severity.

POSSIBLE BENEFITS

May be of great help to migraine sufferers, reducing the number of headaches.

May reduce severity of migraine symptoms, including nausea, vomiting, and head pain.

How to Use It

ORALLY

CAPSULES:
Take 1 up to 3 times daily.

PERSONAL ADVICE

It may take several months before migraine sufferers notice an improvement, but it is well worth the wait. It seems to work in about 80 percent of all cases as a preventive in migraine headaches.

CAUTION

Some people taking feverfew have developed mouth ulcers. If this occurs, discontinue use.

FO-TI

(*Polygonum multiforum*)

FACTS

Known as ho shou wu in China, this herb is used primarily as a rejuvenating tonic. The Chinese claim that fo-ti can prevent hair from going gray as well as preventing other signs of premature aging. It is also believed to increase fertility and maintain strength and vigor. Animal tests using fo-ti extract show antitumor activity. This herb also appears to protect against heart disease by preventing blood clots and reducing blood pressure.

POSSIBLE BENEFITS

May help slow signs of premature aging.

Used generally as a tonic to maintain health and energy.

Good for heart health.

May help prevent cancer.

How to Use It

ORALLY

CAPSULES:
Take 1 up to 3 times daily.

GARLIC GALA

Since 1979, Gilroy, California, known as the "Garlic Capital of the World," has hosted the Annual Garlic Festival in celebration of the annual garlic harvest. The event, which is held the last weekend in July, is a three-day gourmet food and wine tasting party drawing more than 140,000 garlic fans. Ninety percent of the U.S. garlic crop is grown in Gilroy and its environs. American humorist Will Rogers once described Gilroy as "the only town in America where you can marinate a steak by hanging it on the clothesline."

GARLIC

(*Allium sativum*)

FACTS

Garlic may be the wonder drug of the herbal world. The ancient Egyptians not only worshipped garlic but fed it to their slaves to keep them healthy, for good reason. This amazing herb does everything from aid in the treatment of ear infections to help prevent heart disease and cancer. It has even been used to treat tuberculosis, with good results. Biologist Louis Pasteur put garlic to the test by putting a few cloves in a petri dish full of bacteria. Much to his surprise, he discovered that garlic could indeed kill troublesome microorganisms.

In the 1950s, Dr. Albert Schweitzer used garlic to treat cholera, typhus, and amebic dysentery while working as a missionary in Africa. During both world wars, before the availability of antibiotics, garlic was used on the battlefield to disinfect wounds and prevent gangrene. In fact, the Soviet army relied so heavily on garlic that it earned the name "Russian penicillin."

Garlic is also used as an anticoagulant to resolve fresh blood clots and has been shown to lower cholesterol while increasing the level of beneficial HDLs (high-density lipoproteins), the so-called good cholesterol. Garlic also lowers blood pressure. In fact, according to a study published in *Atherosclerosis* when patients with hyperlipoproteinemia ate garlic, blood pressure declined along with levels of LDL (low-density lipoprotein) and fibrinogen. An added bonus was that anticlotting factor levels increased, reducing the risk of blood clots.

There is evidence that garlic can affect the mortality rate of heart attack victims. Researcher Arun Noria at Tagore Medical College in Udaipur, India, monitored 432 heart attack survivors for three years. Half the group drank the juice of six to ten garlic cloves each day. The other half drank a garlic-scented placebo. The garlic eaters experienced 32 percent fewer recurrent heart attacks, and 45 percent fewer deaths.

Hippocrates (460 B.C.) is believed to have used garlic to treat uterine cancer. We now know that garlic is toxic to some tumor cells and is being investigated by the National Cancer Institute (NCI) for its cancer-inhibiting properties. According to a recent NCI study of four thousand people from regions of Italy and China, those who recalled eating diets high in garlic and other alliums, including onions, had a substantially lower incidence of stomach cancer than those who abstained from this pungent herb. Garlic oil can relieve earaches and can help heal minor skin disorders. On top of everything else, garlic is good for indigestion.

POSSIBLE BENEFITS

Helps prevent heart disease by reducing blood pressure and blood lipids.

Helps fight infection.

Can destroy some types of cancer cells.

Excellent digestive aid.

Relieves gas.

How to Use It

ORALLY

CAPSULES:
Aged, odorless garlic is the preferred form in capsules. Take 1 capsule up to 3 times daily.
CLOVES:
Stir-frying the cloves for a few minutes will help eliminate the garlic breath and aftertaste. Two to three cooked cloves daily will reap maximum benefits.

EXTERNALLY

OIL:
Put a few drops of garlic oil (from capsules) in ear for earache. For sprains, aches, and minor skin disorders, rub it directly on affected areas several times daily.

CAUTION

Eating 10 or more raw garlic cloves a day can be toxic and in some cases can trigger an allergic reaction. Garlic should not be used by women who are breast-feeding because it can pass to the breast milk and cause colic in infants.

PERSONAL ADVICE

As research about this amazing herb becomes known to the public, I predict that a new line of odorless, garlic-fortified cereals and beverages will become very popular.

THE GREAT GARLIC MYSTERY

During the Great Plague epidemic, some herbalists avoided this deadly disease by eating large amounts of garlic and wearing garlic strands around their necks. To this day, we don't know whether garlic's antibiotic properties protected these people against plague, or whether the foul stench of the herb discouraged others from getting close enough to spread their infection.

GINGER

(*Zangiber officinale*)

FACTS

Remember when your mother used to give you ginger ale when you felt nauseous? She knew what she was doing. Ginger is a time-proven remedy for upset stomach, indigestion, and cramps. The Chinese have been using ginger for more than two thousand years. The Japanese serve ginger slices between sushi courses to clear the palate and aid digestion. Grated ginger combined with olive oil is an old-fashioned but quite effective remedy for dandruff. (Apply to scalp before you shampoo.) A few drops of this oil can be warmed and used in the ear to soothe earaches. Dr. Albert Leung, a pharmacognosist and renowned expert in Chinese medicine, has recently discovered a new use for gingerroot from the *Journal of New Chinese Medicine*. According to the medical journal, the juice of fresh, crushed gingerroot is an excellent treatment for minor burns and skin inflammations.

POSSIBLE BENEFITS

Calms an upset stomach.

Safe remedy for "morning sickness," a common condition suffered by half of all pregnant women. (Other commercial antinauseants should not be used during pregnancy because of the possibility that they may cross the placenta and adversely affect the fetus.)

Eases cold symptoms.

Soothes and promotes healing of minor burns and skin inflammations.

How to Use It

ORALLY

CAPSULES:
Take 1 up to 3 times daily to relieve symptoms.
EXTRACT:
Mix 15 drops of extract in warm water. This drink can be taken up to 3 times daily.

EXTERNALLY

Mix 15 drops extract in cup of warm vegetable oil. Mash fresh gingerroot, soak in cotton ball, and apply juice directly to inflamed area.

PERSONAL ADVICE

I was discussing certain herbs on a Los Angeles talk show when the host complained that the early-morning drive to the studio—down the steep, winding roads of the Holly-wood Hills—left him feeling nauseous. I suggested that he try gingerroot capsules. It worked. The next day he spent a full five minutes on the show talking about the wonders of this "newfound" remedy for motion sickness!

GINKGO TREE

(*Ginkgo biloba*)

FACTS

For more than five thousand years, Chinese herbalists have recommended this ancient remedy for coughs, asthma, and inflammations due to allergies. Although the ginkgo tree dates back more than two hundred million years—some live as long as four thousand years—we are just beginning to understand its medicinal value. Ginkgo is one of the most well-researched herbs in the world. Most of the research is being done in France and other European countries where ginkgo is a commonly pre-scribed drug.

Ginkgo exerts a positive effect on the vascular system, the body's vast network of blood vessels that delivers blood and oxygen to various organ systems. Recent stud-ies of ginkgo extract show that it increases blood flow to the brain and lower extremities. Ginkgo has been shown to improve memory and to relieve signs of senility, prob-ably due to the increased blood flow to the brain. It also helps prevent blood clots and has been used quite suc-cessfully for problems related to poor circulation, such as phlebitis (inflammation of a vein) and diabetic peripheral vascular disease.

Other studies show that patients suffering from vertigo and tinnitus, or ringing in the ears, experienced dramatic improvement after taking ginkgo due to increased blood flow to the inner ear. Studies also show that ginkgo is an antioxidant, which means that it slows the formation of compounds called free radicals, which are believed to be responsible for premature aging, cancer, and other ills. The nut of the tree makes an excellent expectorant and may provide relief for asthma and allergy sufferers. In 1988, Dr. Elias J. Corey, professor of chemistry at Harvard University, synthesized a ginkgo compound called ginkgolide B, thus increasing the commercial possibilities for this herb in the United States. Among other things, ginkgolide B is being investigated as a potential drug to prevent the rejection of transplanted organs. Researchers are hopeful that it may one day spawn new drugs for asthma and toxic shock syndrome.

POSSIBLE BENEFITS

Improves circulation throughout the body.

Improves mental functioning and the ability to concentrate.

Relieves symptoms of tinnitus such as "ringing in the ears" and vertigo.

May slow aging process.

May help prevent cancer.

May be useful to relieve symptoms of Alzheimer's disease.

Successfully used to treat hemorrhoids in Europe.

How to Use It

ORALLY

CAPSULES OR TABLETS:
Take 40-mg capsules or tablets 3 times daily.

PERSONAL ADVICE

Long-term use is believed to be safe. No known serious side effects have been reported.

GINSENG
(*Panax ginseng*)

FACTS

Ginseng—or len seng in Mandarin—literally means "root of man," so named because the root of this plant resembles the shape of a human body. For the past two decades, ginseng has been touted as a "wonder herb." Many athletes swear that it gives them the competitive edge. Women drink it to alleviate hot flashes and some of the more unpleasant signs of menopause. And millions of others use it as a stimulant and a tonic. Indeed, the reverence in which some hold ginseng is reflected in its botanical name *panax*, which is derived from the Greek word for panacea.

Although we may credit ourselves with discovering this herb, in reality, the Chinese have been using it for more than five thousand years! Ginseng was mentioned in the *Shennong Herbal* (compiled between the first and second centuries B.C.) as a "superior drug" suitable for long-term use without toxic effects. The Chinese were referring to panax ginseng, a variety grown in China. Today, there are three different herbs that fall under the label ginseng. In addition to panax, American ginseng or *Panax quinquefolius* (see page 108) is very popular in China. What is called Siberian ginseng or *Eleutherococcus senticosus* (see page 110) is technically not ginseng at all, but has many of the same properties of ginseng and is therefore used the same way. Although all forms of ginseng have similar properties, there are some subtle differences.

Western interest in ginseng began in the 1960s, when researchers in China, the Soviet Union, Japan, and other European countries began to take a serious look at this herb. In 1969, Soviet scientist I. I. Brekhman, Ph.D., reported that Soviet soldiers who took ginseng extract were able to run faster in a 3-kilometer race than another group given a placebo. Dr. Brekhman was the first to call ginseng an adaptogen, which he described as basically any substance that enables the body to better cope with stress. According to Dr. Brekhman, an adaptogen has the unique ability of being able to normalize body functions. For instance, if blood sugar levels drop too low, or if blood pressure climbs too high, an adaptogen will bring back the body to normal levels. In his writings, Dr. Brekhman has noted that adaptogens work best on people who are neither in peak condition nor in poor health. Rather, they appear to do the most for people who fall somewhere in between those two extremes.

Studies in Japan showed that mice who were fed ginseng learned to perform tasks at a faster rate and made fewer mistakes after taking ginseng. In the 1970s, Japanese researchers found that rats who were fed a high-cholesterol diet showed a drop in cholesterol—especially LDL, or "bad" cholesterol—and a rise in beneficial HDL cholesterol after being given ginseng. A recent study at the Defense Institute of Physiology and Allied Sciences in Delhi, India, showed that rats given ginseng were better able to endure high altitudes and cold temperatures than control rats. Another study at Japan's Kanazawa University found that unpurified saponins from panax ginseng not only inhibited the growth of cancer cells but actually converted the diseased cells into normal cells. Undoubtedly, further studies will be done to determine if some form of ginseng can be used as a cancer treatment.

There have been very few studies of ginseng done in the United States. One famous negative report published in the *Journal of the American Medical Association* described the so-called Ginseng Abuse Syndrome. The article said that heavy users of ginseng were subject to hypertension, nervousness, and insomnia, among other ills. The study, however, included people who took all forms of ginseng—root, powder, extract—as well as those who abused ginseng by injecting it into their veins. The article did not differentiate between caffeine users and noncaffeine users—another substance that could cause similar effects—and is considered by knowledgeable herbal researchers to be completely off-base.

Long before ginseng was studied by the scientific community, Chinese healers were prescribing ginseng to normalize blood pressure, improve blood circulation, and prevent heart disease, among other things. For centuries, ginseng has been purported to be an aphrodisiac, although this claim has never been seriously studied. Many people who take ginseng do find that it has a stimulating effect on the body, increasing their energy and stamina. Ginseng is believed to increase estrogen levels in women and therefore is often recommended for menopausal symptoms caused by a drop in estrogen production. The main active ingredients in ginseng are called ginsenosides. The higher the quantity of ginsenosides, the better the quality of the ginseng.

POSSIBLE BENEFITS

Increases physical and mental endurance.

Helps the body adjust to stressful situations.

Normalizes body functions.

Reduces cholesterol.

Increases energy.

May help reduce discomfort caused by menopause.

May inhibit growth of cancerous tumors.

May enhance sexual desire.

How to Use It

ORALLY

CAPSULES:
   Take 1 up to 3 times daily.
TEA:
   Drink 1 cup daily.
POWDER:
   Mix 5 to 10 grams in liquid daily.

CAUTION

Some people may find panax ginseng too stimulating, especially if used before bedtime. Therefore, use early in the day. High doses may make you feel jittery. Do not exceed 5 to 10 grams daily. In rare cases, some people may develop headaches or high blood pressure from panax ginseng. If you have high blood pressure, check with your doctor before using this product. Take ginseng one hour before or after eating. Vitamin C can interfere with the absorption of ginseng. If you take a vitamin C supplement, wait two hours before or after taking ginseng to do so. In rare cases, ginseng can cause vaginal bleeding in menopausal women, which isn't dangerous but could be mistaken as a symptom of uterine cancer. If you experience any vaginal bleeding, however, be sure to notify your doctor, and be sure to tell him or her that you are taking ginseng.

PERSONAL ADVICE

There are two types of ginseng—red and white—which reflect differences in the processing of the root. White ginseng is simply cleaned and dried; thus, it retains its natural white color. Red ginseng is steamed with a solution of herbs and is considered of superior quality. There have been many reports of diluted or adulterated ginseng products. Your best bet is to buy standardized, guaranteed potency ginseng from a reputable company. In addition, keep in mind that the ginseng-flavored soft drinks that are sold in many health food stores do not offer any of the benefits of true ginseng.

AMERICAN GINSENG

(*Panax quinquefolius*)

FACTS

You may think of Wisconsin as the cheese basket of the country, but it is internationally known for another export—ginseng. In fact, Wisconsin-grown ginseng is highly valued throughout the Orient. Although it is very similar to panax ginseng, and offers many of the same benefits, Chinese herbalists believe that it is somewhat milder and perhaps less stimulating. They often prescribe American ginseng for times of acute stress, such as after a long illness. Native American Indians have used the root of this plant to relieve vomiting and nausea. Some tribes used it in their love potions. American colonists began using ginseng in the early 1700s. The Eccletics, nineteenth-century physicians who rejected synthetic drugs in favor of plant medicines, recommended American ginseng as a stimulant and aphrodisiac.

POSSIBLE BENEFITS

Helps body adapt to stress.

Normalizes body functions.

Works as a mild stimulant.

Enhances physical and mental performance.

Reduces cholesterol.

May inhibit growth of cancerous tumors.

How to Use It

ORALLY

CAPSULES:
   Take 1 up to 3 times daily.
POWDER:
   Mix 1 to 2 teaspoons in warm liquid daily.
TEA:
   Drink 1 cup daily.

SIBERIAN GINSENG
(*Eleutherococcus senticosus*)

FACTS

If Oriental and American ginseng are first cousins in the plant world, Siberian ginseng is a distant relative with a remarkable resemblance to its famous kin. The active chemical ingredients are called eleutherosides. Grown in Siberia, this herb is believed to relieve physical and mental stress and has been used to treat bronchitis and chronic lung ailments. Similar to true ginseng, it normalizes blood pressure and reduces blood cholesterol. Studies of Siberian ginseng by I. I. Brekhman show that, like members of the panax family, it can increase stamina. In fact, Siberian ginseng is routinely used by Russian athletes.

POSSIBLE BENEFITS

Helps body withstand stress.

Improves mental alertness.

Helps cure colds and infections.

Improves overall health.

Helps prevent heart disease by reducing cholesterol and blood pressure.

How to Use It

ORALLY

CAPSULES:
  Take 1 up to 3 times daily.
EXTRACT:
  Mix 5 to 10 drops in warm liquid daily.
LIQUID:
  Take 1 teaspoon up to 3 times daily.

PERSONAL ADVICE

Chinese healers believe that Siberian ginseng is one of the best remedies for insomnia.

JUST WILD ABOUT SAFFRON?

Saffron is the world's most expensive spice (it retails for about forty dollars an ounce!) and no wonder. It takes 50,000 stigmata—a small part of the pistil of the flower—to make a mere 4 ounces of this precious spice. At one time, this herb was highly regarded for its medicinal properties. In 1597, English herbalist John Gerard wrote, "For those at death's doure and almost past breathing, saffron bringeth breath again." Today, saffron is used primarily in cooking by those who can afford it.

GOLDENSEAL

(Hydrastis canadensis)

FACTS

One of the oldest recorded remedies, goldenseal is a broad-spectrum herb that is still extremely popular. Discovered by the aborigines of northern Australia, goldenseal grows freely in the eastern United States and is being cultivated in the West. Long before antibiotics, preparations from this versatile plant were used as a treatment for gonorrhea and syphilis. Today, goldenseal is used to treat symptoms of colds and flu, as well as congestion due to inflammation of the mucous membranes. It is also an excellent laxative and can reduce irritation due to hemorrhoids. This herb is routinely used for female complaints such as vaginitis. A douche of goldenseal can help relieve fungal infections such as candida. Rubbed on the skin, goldenseal tea is a folk remedy for skin ailments including eczema, ringworm, and other inflammations. Used externally, it is an excellent antiseptic and can also soothe irritated gums and canker sores. Combined with myrrh, another "Hot Hundred" herb, goldenseal has been used to treat stomach ulcers.

POSSIBLE BENEFITS

Antiinflammatory action can soothe irritated mucous membranes.

Relieves symptoms of colds and flu.

Aids indigestion and constipation.

Good for skin inflammations such as eczema.

Mouthwash can help prevent gum disease.

Good douche for vaginal infections.

Relieves discomfort caused by ulcers when used with myrrh.

How to Use It

ORALLY

CAPSULES:
Take 1 to 2, up to 3 times daily.
EXTRACT:
Mix 5 to 10 drops in liquid up to 3 times daily.
POWDER:
1 teaspoon can be dissolved in 1 pint of hot water. Let stand until cool. Take 1 to 2 teaspoons for 3 to 6 times daily.

EXTERNALLY

DOUCHE:
Dissolve 1 tablespoon of powder in warm water. Let cool. Douche every 3 days for up to 2 weeks.

CAUTION

This herb can raise blood pressure and should not be used by anyone with a history of high blood pressure. Do not use during pregnancy. Do not use for more than two weeks at a time. Eating the fresh plant can cause inflammation of the mucous tissue.

GOTU KOLA
(*Centella Asiatica*)

FACTS

This herb was probably first used in India, where it is part of *Ayurveda*, the traditional herbal medicine. It was also mentioned in the *Shennong Herbal* compiled in China about two thousand years ago. In recent years, it has become popular in the West as a nerve tonic to promote relaxation and to enhance memory. Indian healers used this herb to treat skin inflammations and as a mild diuretic. Oriental healers relied on gotu kola to treat emotional disorders such as depression that may be rooted in physical problems. It has also been used to bring down a fever and to relieve congestion due to colds and upper respiratory infections.

Recent studies show that gotu kola has a positive effect on the circulatory system: It seems to improve the flow of blood throughout the body by strengthening the veins and capillaries. It has been used successfully to treat phlebitis (inflammation of the veins) as well as leg cramps, swelling of the legs, and "heaviness" or tingling in the legs. It has been shown to be particularly useful for people who are inactive or confined to bed due to illness. Proponents of the herb also believe that its beneficial effect on circulation may help improve memory and brain function.

This herb also has an important role in gynecology. It has been used successfully to promote healing after episiotomy, a surgical incision of the vulva performed to prevent tearing during childbirth. In fact, in one study reported in a French medical journal in 1966, women treated with gotu kola after childbirth healed more rapidly than those given standard treatment.

POSSIBLE BENEFITS

May help improve memory.

Has a calming effect on the body.

Good expectorant—can eliminate congestion due to colds.

Promotes healing after childbirth.

Improves circulation.

Reduces pain and swelling due to phlebitis.

How to Use It

ORALLY

CAPSULES:
Take 1 up to 3 times daily.
EXTRACT:
Mix 5 to 10 drops in liquid. Take 3 times daily.

CAUTION

Do not use during pregnancy. One manufacturer cautions that this herb should not be used by anyone with an overactive thyroid.

HAWTHORNE BERRIES

(*Crataegus oxyacantha*)

FACTS

Long used to treat digestive problems and insomnia, in the late nineteenth century European physicians discovered that the berries from the hawthorne tree were also a cardiotonic. Hawthorne is rich in bioflavonoids, compounds that are essential for vitamin C function and that also help strengthen blood vessels. This herb benefits the heart in many ways. It works as a vasodilator, that is, it increases the flow of blood and oxygen to the heart. It also lowers blood pressure, thus reducing the work required by the heart to pump blood throughout the body. At the same time, it helps strengthen the heart muscle. It also works as a diuretic, helping to rid the body of excess salt and water.

POSSIBLE BENEFITS

Enhances cardiovascular health.

Improves circulation.

How to Use It

ORALLY

CAPSULES:
Take 1 up to 3 times daily.

CAUTION

Although most hawthorne preparations are safe, this herb is also available in a highly concentrated form that should be used only under medical supervision.

HOPS
(*Humulus lupulus*)

FACTS

Despite its name, hops has a calming effect on the body. It is used to relieve gas and cramps (it soothes muscle spasms) and can stimulate the appetite. Hops was originally used in ale as a preservative. For an old-time cure for insomnia, sprinkle hops with alcohol, put it in a pillowcase, and sleep on it.

POSSIBLE BENEFITS

Calms you down.

Relieves indigestion.

An old-time pain reliever.

A good after-dinner tea.

How to Use It

ORALLY

CAPSULES:
Take 1 up to 3 times daily.
DRIED HERB:
Mix 1 teaspoon in ½ cup of warm water. Drink 1 cup daily.

HOREHOUND

(Marrubium vulgare)

FACTS

This is the herb to keep on hand when you have a bad cough due to a cold or bronchitis. It is not only an excellent expectorant but it promotes sweating, which can help break a fever. A mild stimulant, horehound can help relieve the dragged-out, sluggish feeling that often accompanies a bad cold. It is also good for the digestion.

POSSIBLE BENEFITS

Relieves symptoms of coughs and colds.

Rids body of excess water weight.

Promotes sweating, helps cool off the body.

How to Use It

ORALLY

EXTRACT:
For coughs, a tea made from 10 to 40 drops of extract in warm water works best. Use up to 3 times daily.

HORSE CHESTNUT

(Aesculus hippocastum)

FACTS

Although traditionally used as a remedy to bring down a fever and relieve cold symptoms, horse chestnut is being rediscovered in Europe for its ability to reduce swelling of varicose veins and soothe hemorrhoids. Horse chestnut extract has also been used as a sunscreen. According to folklore, carrying around the fruit of this tree in your pocket can prevent and cure arthritis. Many herbalists predict that as the baby boomers approach middle age, horse chestnut will soon enjoy new popularity in the United States.

POSSIBLE BENEFITS

A vagotonic, it strengthens and tones veins.

Soothes irritated varicose veins.

Promotes sweating—can help break a fever.

How to Use It

EXTERNALLY

Commercial preparations for external use are widely available in Europe, but may be difficult to come by in the United States. To make your own, mix ½ teaspoon of horse chestnut powder in 16 ounces of water. Apply mixture gently on varicose veins and hemorrhoids. Do not rub hard—this could cause further irritation.

HORSERADISH

(*Armoracia lapathifolia*)

FACTS

The flavor of the horseradish root is so bitter that it brings tears to the eyes, which is why it is included in the traditional Passover meal to commemorate the suffering of the Jews under Pharaoh's rule. It is also an excellent diuretic and is good for digestion. Herbalists combine horseradish with honey for coughs and asthma. Externally, it can be used to alleviate the pain and stiffness caused by rheumatism.

POSSIBLE BENEFITS

Good expectorant, soothing for respiratory problems.

May help relieve rheumatism by stimulating blood flow to inflamed joints.

How to Use It

ORALLY

GRATED ROOT:
Mix grated root with honey and warm water. Use daily for bad cough. (It may not taste very good, but it is very effective.)
TABLETS:
Take 1 up to 3 times daily.

EXTERNALLY

Fresh horseradish can be made into a poultice by adding it to cornstarch. Apply to affected areas in a gauze bandage.

CAUTION

Do not take large quantities at one time—it could cause diarrhea and excessive sweating.

PERSONAL ADVICE

It's best to use the fresh product if it is available at your grocery store or herb store.

HORSETAIL

(Equisetum arvense)

FACTS

Long used by herbal healers in Europe and China, horsetail—also known as silica—is rich in nutrients, including silicon. Horsetail facilitates the absorption of calcium by the body, which nourishes nails, skin, hair, bones, and the body's connective tissue. This herb helps eliminate excess oil from skin and hair and is believed to make individual hair strands stronger, thicker, and more resilient.

POSSIBLE BENEFITS

Good conditioner for nails and hair.

Helps eliminate white spots from nails.

Controls excess oil on skin.

Helps strengthen bones.

How to Use It

ORALLY

CAPSULES OR TABLETS:
Take 1 up to 3 times daily

EXTERNALLY

Horsetail is used in many herbal beauty products for skin, nails, and hair.

HYSSOP

(*Hyssopus officinalis*)

FACTS

This herb is useful to treat a bad cold, cough, and stuffy nose of a bad cold. It will help relieve the heavy, congested feeling in the head and chest. Studies show that it has antiviral properties and can be useful in treating cold sores. It can also be used for indigestion.

POSSIBLE BENEFITS

Good expectorant for coughs and cold.

Relieves gas.

Improves the appetite.

Good gargle for sore throat.

How to Use It

ORALLY

DRIED HERB:
Mix 1 teaspoon in ½ cup warm water. Drink up to 3 times daily for cough. Gargle up to 3 times daily for sore throats and cold sores.

CAUTION

Do not take for more than two weeks without seeking medical advice.

JASMINE

(*Jasminum officinale*)

FACTS

For centuries, the flowers from the jasmine plant have been brewed into a tea that is both delicious and relaxing. Many commercial jasmine teas are available today. According to folklore, the oil from this flower can be sexually arousing if rubbed on the body.

POSSIBLE BENEFITS

Calms you down.

Good after-dinner drink.

Possible aphrodisiac.

How to Use It

ORALLY

TEA:
Drink 1 cup daily.

JUNIPER BERRIES

(Juniperus communis)

FACTS

In the 1500s, a Dutch pharmacist used juniper berries to create a new, inexpensive diuretic that he called gin. The drink caught on for other reasons, and the juniper berry is now just one of several ingredients. For centuries, juniper has been a folk remedy for urinary tract problems including urinary retention and gallstones. It has also been used successfully to treat gout, a condition marked by painful inflammation of the joints caused by deposits of uric acid and a high uric acid content in the blood. The berry is good for digestion and can help eliminate gas and cramps.

POSSIBLE BENEFITS

Relieves urinary tract problems.

Old-time treatment for gout.

Helps improve digestion.

Helps rid the body of excess fluid.

How to Use It

ORALLY

EXTRACT:
    Take 10 to 20 drops up to 3 times daily.
TEA:
    Drink 1 cup up to 3 times daily.

CAUTION

Do not use during pregnancy.

KAVA KAVA
(*Piper methysticum*)

FACTS

Kava kava was first discovered by explorer Captain James Cook, who gave this plant the botanical name of "intoxicating pepper." The root of this plant is made into a popular beverage in Polynesia called Sakau. Herbalists here have traditionally used it as a remedy for nervousness and insomnia. It can also help relieve cramping due to muscle spasms. Kava kava is a mild diuretic.

POSSIBLE BENEFITS

Helps you get a good night's sleep.

Promotes relaxation.

Helps reduce water retention.

How to Use It

ORALLY

EXTRACT:
Mix 10 to 30 drops in juice or water.

CAUTION

Use only occasionally to relieve periods of stress or sleeplessness. Long-term use can cause liver damage.

LADY'S MANTLE

(*Alchemilla vulgaris*)

FACTS

Women in Arab countries believe that this herb restores beauty and youth—needless to say, it is very popular in that part of the world. Traditionally, lady's mantle has been used by Western herbalists topically on wounds to stop bleeding and promote healing. Taken internally, it is used to regulate menstruation and stimulate the appetite. It also makes a soothing douche for mild vaginal irritations. The botanical name, alchemilla, is derived from the word *alchemy*, because the herbs in this family are believed to bring about miraculous cures.

POSSIBLE BENEFITS

Promotes coagulation of blood, stops bleeding.

Promotes menstrual regularity.

Improves appetite.

Reduces vaginal irritation.

How to Use It

ORALLY

TEA:
Put 1 tablespoon of dried herb in hot water (or in tea ball). Strain. Drink 1 cup daily.

EXTERNALLY

EXTRACT:
Dissolve 5 to 10 drops in 16 ounces of water and use as a douche. It can also be applied to wounds.

LICORICE

(Glycyrrhiza globra)

FACTS

Licorice-flavored candy has been a popular confection for centuries. The root of this plant, however, is also highly regarded for its medicinal properties. The *Shennong Herbal,* a list of more than 365 plant drugs compiled in China about two thousand years ago, lists licorice as a "superior" drug, meaning that it can be used over a long period of time with no toxic effects. Culpeper wrote that this herb is "a fine medicine for hoarseness."

More recently, foreign studies show that glycyrrhizin, a saponin found in licorice root, has antiinflammatory, antiviral, and antiallergic properties. Licorice root is soothing for peptic ulcers, bladder ailments, and kidney ailments. It is also a good expectorant. Licorice is a time-honored remedy for arthritis due to its antiinflammatory properties: It stimulates the production of two steroids, cortisone and aldosterone, which help reduce inflammation. The Japanese are investigating glycyrrhetic acid as a possible cancer treatment. In the United States, the National Cancer Institute is investigating triterpenoids, compounds found in licorice root, for their ability to inhibit the growth of cancerous cells and prevent tooth decay.

POSSIBLE BENEFITS

Reduces pain from ulcers.

Useful for urinary tract problems.

Helps break up congestion due to colds.

Soothes sore, hoarse throat.

Reduces pain and stiffness from arthritis.

May help retard growth of certain cancerous tumors.

May help prevent cavities.

How to Use It

ORALLY

CAPSULES:
Take 1 up to 3 times daily.

CAUTION

Do not use if you have high blood pressure. The increased production of aldosterone can result in a rise in blood pressure. In large quantities, licorice can sap potassium from the body, which is extremely dangerous. Licorice candy does not offer the same benefits as preparations made from the root, but can cause an increase in blood pressure.

PERSONAL ADVICE

Women who suffer from premenstrual syndrome (PMS) should not use licorice during PMS time due to its ability to cause water retention or bloating.

LUNGWORT
(*Pulmonaria officinalis*)

FACTS

As its name suggests, this herb is good for coughs, hoarseness, and mild lung problems. It can also be used for diarrhea, which makes it the herb of choice for a stomach virus accompanied by a cough.

POSSIBLE BENEFITS

Good expectorant, breaks up chest congestion.

Can soothe throat irritation.

Helps cure diarrhea.

How to Use It

ORALLY

DRIED HERB:
Mix 1 tablespoon herb in 1 cup hot water. Drink 1 cup daily.

CAUTION

If you have a cough that lasts for more than two weeks, do not try to self-medicate. See a medical professional immediately.

READING BETWEEN THE LINES

The "Doctrine of Signatures," a concept popular in the fifteenth century, espoused that God revealed an herb's medicinal purpose by providing special markings on the plant. There are many herbs that indeed support this theory. For example, the leaves of the lungwort plant, an excellent treatment for upper respiratory infections and lung ailments, have spotted markings that are characteristic of delicate lung tissue. The root of the ginseng plant, an herb reputed to be good for nearly every organ system, resembles the shape of the human body.

MARSHMALLOW

(Althea officinalis)

FACTS

King Charlemagne (A.D. 742–814) insisted that this herb be planted throughout his kingdom to ensure an abundant supply. Perhaps he had ulcers or colitis, because marshmallow is an old-time remedy for gastrointestinal disorders. It is high in mucilage, a substance that when combined with water develops a gel-like consistency. Mucilage can be very soothing to irritated mucous membranes. In fact, about eight hundred years after Charlemagne's death, Culpeper wrote that his son suffered from a disease called the "bloody flux," which the College of Physicians back then called the plague in the guts. Culpeper treated his son by giving him "mallow bruised and boiled both in milk and drink." Two days later, his son was cured. Today, herbalists still use marshmallow to treat ulcers and colitis. It is also highly recommended for the raw, irritated feeling in the throat and chest often caused by bad coughs and bronchitis.

POSSIBLE BENEFITS

Relieves pain caused by ulcers, enteritis, and colitis.

Has a calming effect on the body.

Good expectorant for coughs.

Soothes throat/chest irritation due to coughs and colds.

How to Use It

ORALLY

CAPSULES:
Take 1 up to 3 times daily to relieve symptoms.
DRIED HERB:
Mix 1 tablespoon of dried herb in 8 ounces boiling water. Strain. Drink up to 3 cups of this tea daily to relieve symptoms.

MILK THISTLE
(*Cardus marianus*)

FACTS

Milk thistle is extremely popular in Europe as a tonic for the liver, the body's second largest organ. This herb contains a flavonoid called silymarin that has been shown to have a direct effect on liver cells. (Known as vitamin P, flavonoids are substances found in plants that often work in conjunction with vitamin C and offer many other health benefits.) Often referred to as the body's "chemical factory," the liver plays a critical role in maintaining good health. It produces bile, which is necessary for the breakdown of fats. It detoxifies poisons that enter our bloodstream, such as nicotine, alcohol, and pollutants such as carbon monoxide: It breaks them down from potentially lethal substances into those that are less destructive to our bodies. The liver is also the site where vitamins A, D, E, and K are stored. Numerous European studies show that this herb enhances overall liver function, as well as stimulates the production of new liver cells.

POSSIBLE BENEFITS

Rejuvenates the liver.

Increases production of bile used for breakdown of fats.

How to Use It

ORALLY

CAPSULES:
Take 1 capsule for 3 times daily.

PERSONAL ADVICE

This herb can be beneficial for those suffering from hepatitis or inflammation of the liver. It is also useful for people who have developed cirrhosis of the liver, a condition often caused by excessive alcohol intake. I also recommend it for anyone who smokes or who is exposed to pollutants in the workplace.

MULLEIN

(*Verbascum thapsus*)

FACTS

This herb is an old-time remedy for bronchitis and dry, unproductive coughs. It is a good expectorant, and in the process of clearing out the congestion, it also soothes irritation in the throat and bronchial passages. An antispasmodic, mullein can relieve stomach cramps and help control diarrhea.

POSSIBLE BENEFITS

Reduces irritation due to coughs and bronchitis.

Helps relieve gastrointestinal stress.

How to Use It

ORALLY

DRIED HERB:
Mix 1 tablespoon of herb in 8 ounces warm water. Drink 1 to 2 cups tea daily.
EXTRACT:
Mix 25 to 40 drops in liquid. Drink 3 to 4 times daily for coughs.

PERSONAL ADVICE

This is a good herb to have handy for a flu accompanied by stomach cramps and a chest cold. For those of you who can find the actual plant, the leaves can be boiled in water and the steam can be inhaled to relieve coughs and congestion.

MYRRH

(*Commiphora myrrha*)

And when they came into the house, they saw the young child with Mary his mother, and fell down, and worshipped him: and when they had opened their treasures, they presented unto him gifts; gold, and frankincense, and myrrh.

—ST. MATTHEW 2:11

FACTS

Since ancient times, the resin or gum of the myrrh plant has been used as a mouthwash for sores in the mouth and throat. It is also a popular treatment for irritated and infected gums. In addition, myrrh may help relieve upper respiratory infections due to coughs and cold. It not only soothes irritated bronchial passages but studies suggest that myrrh stimulates the body's immune system, increasing resistance to infection. According to the Bible, both Kings David and Solomon sang the praises of this herb, which was also used by Moses in Jewish ceremonial rites. Myrrh was so highly regarded, according to scripture, that it was presented to the infant Jesus by the three wise men.

POSSIBLE BENEFITS

Excellent antiseptic and mouthwash.

Promotes healing of mouth sores.

Strengthens "spongy" or soft gums.

Good for coughs and colds.

Good for stomach flu.

133

How to Use It

ORALLY

DRIED HERB:
Mix 1 tablespoon herb to 8 ounces warm water. Drink
1 cup tea daily for colds.
EXTRACT:
Mix 2 to 5 drops in water for an excellent mouthwash.

CAUTION

Very high doses over a long period of time can be dangerous. Therefore, do not exceed recommended dose. Do not
use if you are pregnant or have kidney disease without
first checking with your physician.

NETTLE
(*Urtica dioica*)

FACTS

Nettle is a well-known folk remedy for hayfever and other
allergies. It helps relieve inflammation caused by allergic
reactions and clears congestion in the nose and chest. According to a recent study conducted at the National College of Naturopathic Medicine, 57 percent of the 69
patients who finished the trial found nettle to be moderately or highly effective in relieving allergy symptoms.
Out of this group, half found it to be as good or better than
other hayfever medications they had previously taken.
Nettle is also a good herb for women. It is used for vaginal
infections such as candida (yeast infection) and to control

excessive menstrual flow. Rich in iron and vitamin C, nettle can help prevent anemia. Nettle also increases milk production in nursing mothers. In animal studies, nettle has been shown to lower blood sugar, which could help prevent diabetes.

POSSIBLE BENEFITS

Alleviates stuffy nose, watery eyes, and other symptoms of hayfever.

Helps cure vaginal infections.

Helps normalize menstrual flow.

Lowers blood sugar.

Provides iron for the production of red blood cells.

How to Use It

ORALLY

CAPSULES:
Take 1 to 2 capsules daily, up to 4 times per day for hayfever (for a total of 8 capsules).
DRIED HERB:
Mix 1 tablespoon in 8 ounces warm water. Drink 1 cup tea daily for hemorrhoids.
EXTRACT:
Mix 5 to 10 drops in liquid daily.

CAUTION

Do not eat uncooked plants—they can cause kidney damage and symptoms of poisoning. Handle plants with care. The bristly hairs act like tiny hypodermic needles, injecting an irritant under the skin.

OAT FIBER
(Avena sativa)

FACTS

Long before breakfast meant a bowl of sugar-coated, artificially flavored cereal, our "less enlightened" ancestors thrived on whole grains such as oatmeal. The grain from the oat plant is not only nutritious but we now know that oat fiber serves another important purpose: It is one of the most effective ways to reduce serum cholesterol. Rich in a gum called beta glucam, 2 to 3 ounces of oat fiber per day in a low-fat diet can reduce cholesterol by 5 to 10 percent. Oat extract is a natural relaxant. It is also excellent for indigestion. No part of the oat plant need go to waste: The dried coarse stem or straw can be used in baths to soothe hemorrhoids and to revitalize sore, aching feet.

POSSIBLE BENEFITS

Good for gas and upset stomach.

Helps prevent heart disease by reducing cholesterol.

Good source of vitamin B.

Good for skin and hemorrhoids.

Extract has a calming effect on the body.

How to Use It

ORALLY

Eat foods rich in oat fiber.
EXTRACT:
For indigestion, take 10 to 20 drops up to 3 times daily to relieve symptoms.

EXTERNALLY

The straw is used in external preparations in baths, sitz baths for hemorrhoids, and footbaths.

PERSONAL ADVICE

Gradually increase the amount of oat bran you eat every day, giving your body time to adjust to the change in diet. If you take in too much at once, you may suffer from cramps and gas.

OLIVE

(Olea europaea)

FACTS

Since biblical times, the branch from the olive tree has been a symbol for peace and prosperity. It is also an extremely useful plant. The leaves have been used to reduce fever and as a mild tranquilizer. The precious oil is an excellent laxative. It also stimulates the production of bile in the liver. Externally, it can be used to soothe insect bites, itching, and bruises. Warm olive oil makes a terrific conditioner for dry hair and scalp. Olive oil, high in monounsaturated fats, has received attention recently because of its ability to reduce "bad" cholesterol in the blood—LDLs—without reducing good cholesterol—HDLs. Studies show that people who eat diets high in olive oil have a lower incidence of heart disease than those who eat diets high in other forms of fat. To prevent heart disease, nutritionists recommend that you limit your daily intake of fat calories to 30 percent of your total daily caloric intake, and that about 10 to 15 percent should be in the form of monounsaturates such as olive oil.

POSSIBLE BENEFITS

Relieves constipation by promoting contraction of the bowels.

Good for skin irritations.

Reduces cholesterol.

Good hair "tonic" for dry scalp.

How to Use It

ORALLY

OIL:
For laxative, drink 1 to 2 ounces straight-up per day. To reduce cholesterol, substitute 1 to 2 tablespoons of olive oil for other fat in cooking or on salad daily.

EXTERNALLY

Rub on affected areas.

CAUTION

Do not use as a laxative during pregnancy.

ONION
(*Allium cepa*)

FACTS

The everyday onion is one of the oldest and most versatile remedies. Long before commercial cold remedies, herbalists used a syrup made from the juice of one onion mixed with honey to alleviate congestion. Culpeper recommends it "to help an inveterate cough, and expectorate tough phlegm." I've tried it myself, and the stuff works as well as many over-the-counter cough medicines without some of the unpleasant side effects, like drowsiness or nervousness. Onion is also excellent for indigestion.

A roasted onion can be used as a poultice for earaches. Onion is believed to be a natural source of energy, and some people swear that an onion a day can prevent hair loss. Applied directly to the skin, onion has special healing properties. Salted onions are useful for troublesome warts. Onion juice rubbed between the toes 2 to 3 times daily can cure athlete's foot. A mixture of 1 to 2 teaspoons onion juice with 1 teaspoon vinegar can fade unsightly liver spots or dark blemishes.

An onion a day may also keep the cardiologist away. Studies show that people who eat a medium-sized onion daily can lower their overall cholesterol and raise their HDL, or "good" cholesterol. Onion has also been shown to lower blood pressure and help prevent blood clots. A recent study by the National Cancer Institute showed that people who eat diets high in allium vegetables such as onion (and garlic) suffer from less stomach cancer than those who don't. According to folklore, onion helps restore sexual potency.

POSSIBLE BENEFITS

Good expectorant.

Relieves symptoms of common cold.

Relieves gas.

Helps prevent heart disease and cancer.

Antifungal—good for warts.

Good antiseptic.

How to Use It

ORALLY

JUICE:
> Take 1 teaspoon for 3 to 4 times daily. To make onion juice, puree one raw onion in a blender or food processor and strain through cheesecloth. Store in the refrigerator. For colds, mix warm juice with 2 teaspoons honey.

FRESH HERB:
> Onions can also be eaten raw.

EXTERNALLY

> Rub juice on warts or between toes to fight athlete's foot. Can be used as antiseptic on skin wounds.

CAUTION

When chopping fresh onions, beware of eye irritation. If you're breast-feeding an infant, stay clear of onions, because they could cause the baby to suffer colic.

PERSONAL ADVICE

Try eating a parsley sprig to avoid "onion breath." Chlorophyll tablets also can help eliminate odor.

PAPAYA
(*Carica papaya*)

FACTS

If you can't get through a day without popping an antacid (or two or three), this is the herb for you. Papaya contains a substance called papain, which is chemically similar to pepsin, an enzyme that helps digest protein in the body. It is a safe and natural digestive aid. I know that it's easy enough to buy an over-the-counter alternative, but it is certainly not any better. In fact, in a lot of ways, it is much worse. If you take too many antacids, you run the risk of the "rebound effect," that is, your body will respond by producing even more acid, which will cause even more gastrointestinal problems. Papaya juice or tablets, however, can be taken freely without any fear of rebounding. The fruit is also delicious and very popular in Hawaii.

POSSIBLE BENEFITS

Aids in the breakdown and metabolism of protein.

Helps relieve indigestion.

How to Use It

ORALLY

JUICE:
   Take 1 teaspoon to 1 tablespoon as needed.
TABLETS:
   Take 1 up to 3 times daily to relieve symptoms.

PERSONAL ADVICE

Papaya is commercially available in a delicious, chewable tablet form. Dried papaya slices are also an excellent way to take advantage of this herb's benefits.

PARSLEY

(Petroselinum sativum)

FACTS

Every night after dinner, my grandmother used to make herself a cup of parsley tea. She'd take a few sprigs of parsley, steep them in hot water for several minutes, and then sip the tea slowly. When I asked her why she did it, she shrugged and said that her grandmother told her to. Her grandmother knew what she was doing. Parsley is a natural antispasmodic—in other words, it's great for the digestion. It relieves gas and is a natural diuretic. It is also a good expectorant and can be used for coughs and asthma. Herbalists used parsley oil to regulate menstruation and induce abortion. Rubbed on the scalp, parsley oil purportedly stimulates hair growth.

POSSIBLE BENEFITS

Helps "settle" the stomach after a meal.

Helps clear congestion due to coughs and colds.

Soothing for asthma.

Parsley oil may induce menstruation.

How to Use It

ORALLY

Eat raw, or steep chopped leaves and stem in hot water. Drink daily.

CAUTION

Pregnant women should not take parsley juice or oil.

PERSONAL ADVICE

This herb is one of the few things that can be eaten raw on the plate. It's a wonderful source of chlorophyll, nature's own breath freshener. Try it after eating onions or garlic.

PASSIONFLOWER

(*Passiflora incarnata*)

FACTS

This herb is one of nature's best tranquilizers. It relieves muscle tension and other manifestations of extreme anxiety. It is especially good for nervous insomnia—the kind that keeps you lying in bed worrying until the wee hours of the morning. Since the tryptophan scare, in which a contaminated batch of this essential amino acid was linked to several deaths, passionflower has become very popular as a safe, natural alternative to help promote a good night's sleep. Herbalists often recommend passionflower for times of extreme emotional upset.

POSSIBLE BENEFITS

Calms you down.

Can relieve headaches due to nervous tension.

Good for muscle spasms due to nerves.

143

How to Use It

ORALLY

EXTRACT:
Mix 15 to 60 drops in liquid as needed daily.

CAUTION

This herb may cause sleepiness in some people and should not be used before driving or operating machinery. Do not take during pregnancy.

THE MARIJUANA STORY

Cannabis (marijuana), the dried, flowering spikes of the hemp plant, is a well-known psychoactive drug that was made into hashish by certain Muslim sects in the Middle Ages. The word *assassin* is derived from the Arab *hashshashin,* which refers to a secret order of Muslims that terrorized the Christian crusaders by committing murder while under the influence of this potent drug.

PAU D'ARCO
(Tabecuia impetiginosa)

FACTS

From Brazil comes the bark of this tree that has numerous health benefits. It's an old-time remedy for candida, athlete's foot, and other annoying fungal infections. Research in South America and the United States shows that lapachol, an extract from the tree's bark, contains active ingredients found to be effective against some forms of cancer. However, lapachol is not considered a viable cancer treatment because tests on humans conducted by the National Cancer Institute indicated that high levels can cause many undesirable side effects. Another study done at the Naval Medical Research Institute in Bethesda, Maryland, in 1974 found that lapachol is quite useful against parasitic infection. Pau d'arco seems to lower blood sugar levels, which may help prevent diabetes. On top of everything else, this herb is reputed to be good for the digestion!

POSSIBLE BENEFITS

Helps cure fungal infections.

Helps fight parasitic infection.

Promotes good digestion.

Lowers blood sugar.

How to Use It

ORALLY

CAPSULES:
   Take 1 up to 3 times daily.
EXTRACT:
   Mix 25 to 40 drops in liquid up to 3 times daily.
TEA:
   Drink 1 cup up to 3 times daily.

PENNYROYAL

(*Hedeoma pulegioides*)

FACTS

Often referred to as the "lung mint," this herb was used to treat coughs and colds. It promotes perspiration, which helps break a fever. American Indians used pennyroyal to relieve menstrual cramps. Herbalists use pennyroyal today to induce menstruation and to treat monthly symptoms associated with premenstrual syndrome (PMS), such as bloating and breast tenderness.

POSSIBLE BENEFITS

Helps promote "productive" cough.

Good to take at onset of cold.

Brings on menstruation.

Relieves PMS and menstrual cramps.

How to Use It

ORALLY

DRIED HERB:
Mix 1 tablespoon with 8 ounces of warm water and take daily.
EXTRACT:
Mix 20 to 60 drops in liquid daily for relief of symptoms.

CAUTION

Back in the days when abortion was illegal, this herb was used to induce abortion. In some cases, it resulted in hemorrhaging and serious complications for the mother. Therefore, it should never be used for this purpose. Today, pennyroyal is one of the herbs used by herbalists to facilitate labor and delivery. It should be used only under the supervision of a knowledgeable practitioner. If you do use this herb, do not exceed the recommended dose and do not take for more than a week at a time.

PERSONAL ADVICE

Pennyroyal oil makes an excellent bug repellent for pets. Put a few drops of the oil directly on the animal.

PEPPERMINT

(*Mentha piperita*)

FACTS

Peppermint is one of the oldest and best-tasting home remedies for indigestion. Studies show that peppermint lessens the amount of time food spends in the stomach by stimulating the gastric lining. It also relaxes the stomach muscles and promotes burping. Peppermint is excellent for heartburn and stomachache. It is also good for nausea and vomiting. Migraine headaches, which are frequently accompanied by nausea, are often relieved by peppermint. This herb has a calming effect on the body and can help soothe a nagging cough.

POSSIBLE BENEFITS

Antispasmodic—good for cramps and stomach pain.

Relieves gas.

Aids in digestion.

Can help reduce sick feeling typical of migraine headaches.

Can help with insomnia.

How to Use It

ORALLY

TEA:
Drink 1 cup daily. Many commercial teas are available.

PERSONAL ADVICE

This is an excellent substitute for regular coffee and tea—and better-tasting too. For a headache, try a strong cup of peppermint tea and lie down for 15 to 20 minutes. I think that it works better than aspirin or acetaminophen. Considering all the things that peppermint can do, no home medicine cabinet should be without it! In drop form, peppermint has been used for centuries for colic in infants and in liquid form for older children. Check with your pediatrician before giving this or any other herb to your child.

PLEURISY ROOT

(*Asclepias tuberosa*)

FACTS

As its name suggests, this herb is used for ailments involving the lungs and upper respiratory problems. It's also good for indigestion and "gassy stomach." Native Americans used this root to treat bronchitis, pneumonia, and diarrhea.

POSSIBLE BENEFITS

Helps clear phlegm from chest.

Good digestive aid.

How to Use It

ORALLY

DRIED HERB:
   Mix 1 tablespoon with 8 ounces warm liquid. Drink 1 cup daily.
EXTRACT:
   Mix 5 to 40 drops in liquid every 3 hours for relief of symptoms.

CAUTION

The fresh root can be dangerous. Use only commercial preparations.

PSYLLIUM
(*Plantago psyllium*)

FACTS

A leading cereal manufacturer recently discovered what herbalists have known for decades: Ground-up seeds from the psyllium plant are one of the highest sources of dietary fiber to be found in any food. For centuries, psyllium has been used to treat ulcers, colitis, and constipation. We now know that it helps clear the body of excess cholesterol: This herb is now touted as a preventive against heart disease. It may also raise the level of beneficial HDLs, the so-called good cholesterol, in the blood.

POSSIBLE BENEFITS

An excellent laxative that offers relief from hemorrhoidal irritation.

May help prevent heart disease.

Good for gastrointestinal irritations.

How to Use It

ORALLY

GROUND SEEDS OR POWDER:
Mix 1 teaspoon in 1 cup liquid, and drink 2 to 3 times daily.

CAUTION

Psyllium can cause allergic reactions in sensitive individuals. If you are highly allergic to many other substances, I recommend that you avoid this one, or certainly check with your allergist before taking it. If you want to include psyllium in your diet, you should start slowly, allowing your body time to get used to the increased fiber. Be patient. In two to three weeks, it will. Too much at one time could cause gassiness and stomach discomfort. It is important to drink 8 to 10 glasses of water throughout the day when you are using this substance to increase its efficiency. If you develop any allergic symptoms, discontinue use. Do not use psyllium to treat an ulcer or colitis without checking with your doctor.

RASPBERRY LEAVES

(Rubus idaeus)

FACTS

Back in the days when midwives were the primary health-care providers to women and "natural" childbirth was the only way to have a baby, the leaf of the raspberry bush was the herb of choice. Women routinely brewed it into a tea to drink during their last two months of pregnancy to tone their uterine muscles for labor and delivery. After birth, raspberry tea was taken for several weeks to help the uterus return to normal. It is also excellent for menstrual cramps. Warm raspberry tea is also soothing for throat irritations and canker sores and is effective against diarrhea.

POSSIBLE BENEFITS

Prepares the uterus for childbirth, may help shorten delivery.

Good for sore throats and fever blisters.

Alleviates menstrual cramps.

How to Use It

ORALLY

DRIED HERB:
Mix 1 teaspoon herb in 1 cup warm water. Drink daily.
EXTRACT:
Mix 15 to 30 drops 3 times daily. Drink warm for best results.
TEA:
Drink 1 cup tea daily.

CAUTION

Do not use during pregnancy until last two months, and then only under the supervision of a qualified health practitioner.

RED CLOVER
(*Trifolium pratense*)

FACTS

Traditionally, the blossoms from this plant were used as a tonic taken in the spring to promote good health and peace of mind. It contains small amounts of silica, choline, calcium, and lecithin—all essential for normal body function. It works as a muscle relaxer and also is a good expectorant. It is an old-time remedy for eczema.

Combined with other herbs, red clover is used to treat cancers and tumors. In the 1940s, this herb received a good deal of notoriety because it was included in herbal healer Harry Hoxsey's anticancer formula, dubbed the "red clover combination." Hoxsey ran a chain of cancer clinics that were under frequent attack by the American Medical Association. At that time, the only legitimate treatments for cancer were surgery or radiation. Although the medical establishment portrayed Hoxsey as a quack, we now know that many of the herbs included in his formula have antitumor properties. Modern research also validates the use of other herbs, such as Madagascar periwinkle for leukemia and Pacific hew for uterine and prostate cancer. Although Hoxsey's formula may not have been a cure-all for cancer, he was a pioneer in incorporating folklore treatments in modern-day cancer therapy.

POSSIBLE BENEFITS

Calms coughs, clears chest of phlegm.

Good for skin inflammations.

Relaxes the body.

Helps fight against cancerous growths.

Improves overall health.

How to Use It

ORALLY

CAPSULES:
Take 1 capsule up to 3 times daily.
EXTRACT:
Mix 10 to 30 drops in warm liquid daily.

CAUTION

Please seek professional help before using this or any other herb to treat tumors and cancer. Any cancer treatment should be done under the supervision of a physician.

ST. JOHN'S WORT
(*Hypericum perforatum*)

FACTS

If you rub the petals of this flower between your fingers, red resin will ooze out, leaving a stain on your hand. Perhaps that is why, according to a legend dating back to the Middle Ages, this plant sprang from John the Baptist's blood when he was beheaded. Through the years, this herb has been used as a mild tranquilizer and as a treatment for depression and insomnia. In fact, recent studies show that it is quite effective for anxiety and emotional problems; unlike many other psychotropic drugs, the patients did not report any side effects. St. John's Wort is also a muscle relaxer that has been used to treat menstrual cramps. It is a good expectorant as well.

In Europe, it is also a popular remedy for gastrointestinal disorders such as gastric ulcers. Externally, it is an antiseptic and a painkiller for burns and irritations. Ointments are also used for rheumatism and sciatica or back pain. This herb has gotten a lot of attention recently after researchers at two of the world's leading medical institutions—New York University and the Weizman Institute of Science in Israel—found that two of its main constituents, hypericin and pseudohypericin, were found to inhibit the growth of retro viruses in animals, including HIV, the AIDS virus. Although the results of these studies are promising, a synthetic form of hypericin is just now being tested on HIV-infected patients. More studies are needed to determine if this herb can be useful against AIDS.

POSSIBLE BENEFITS

Good for anxiety.

Has a calming effect on the body.

Relieves uterine cramping.

Promotes healing of skin wounds.

Helps the body fight viral infection.

How to Use It

ORALLY

EXTRACT:
Mix 10 to 15 drops in liquid daily.

CAUTION

Although there have been no reports of any problems in humans, this herb can be poisonous to cattle. It also causes sensitivity to light, which means that if you use it, you should avoid exposure to the sun.

PERSONAL ADVICE

I would not recommend this herb for long-term use, but I feel that it is safe for short-term use. Although, in many cases, it is safer than some of the medication typically prescribed for anxiety and emotional problems, your best bet is to use this herb under the supervision of a medical professional.

SARSAPARILLA

(*Smilux officinalis*)

FACTS

Since it was brought to Europe from the New World by Spanish traders in the 1600s, there has been a mystique surrounding this controversial herb. Originally, sarsaparilla was used to treat syphilis, but it soon became known as a tonic for male sexual potency. Some herbalists claim that its steroidlike compounds—saponin glycosides—actually contain male hormones. This has never been proven, although these substances appear to stimulate the body's metabolic processes. Because it promotes urination and sweating, sarsaparilla has been touted as a "blood purifier" by old-time herbalists who believed that toxins are released through bodily secretions. At the very least, these properties mean that the herb can be useful in cooling down the body or breaking a fever.

Recently, this herb has been marketed as a "male herb" that can increase muscle mass much the same way as steroids do. There is no evidence to back up this claim. At the turn of the century, the claims for this herb were no less grandiose. In fact, it was sold as a cure-all for nearly every malady known to man (and woman, for that matter!). Because of a lack of sound research, when it comes to sarsaparilla, it's difficult to separate fact from fiction. All we know is that for centuries, different cultures have utilized this herb often in surprisingly similar ways. For example, Europeans used sarsaparilla as an anti-inflammatory for rheumatism, arthritis, and also as a treatment for urinary tract disorders; so did the Chinese. Native Americans also used this herb for urinary problems, arthritis, and as a rejuvenating tonic. In fact, until 1950, sarsaparilla was included in the *U.S. Pharmacopeia*, and was recommended by the U.S. Dispensatory for the treatment of secondary syphilis. Many people today still use sarsaparilla as a tonic.

POSSIBLE BENEFITS

Good diuretic—induces sweating and urination.

Useful for urinary problems.

Relieves swelling and soreness of rheumatism and arthritis.

May enhance physical performance.

How to Use It

ORALLY

CAPSULES:
Take 1 up to 3 times daily.
EXTRACT:
Mix 10 to 30 drops in liquid daily. (For fevers, use warm liquid.)

PERSONAL ADVICE

This herb is being used today by bodybuilders who have told me they have better workouts when they use Smilax (from the botanical name *Smilax officinalis*).

SAW PALMETTO
(Serenoa serrulata)

FACTS

This herb is used to treat coughs due to colds as well as asthma and bronchitis. It is also reputed to be beneficial for the reproductive organs of both sexes, working as an aphrodisiac and a tonic. In fact, herbalists use it to treat "honeymoon cystitis"—irritations due to excessive sexual activity. Although the FDA does not recognize saw palmetto as an effective drug, in Germany it is used in over-the-counter treatments for benign prostate enlargement, a condition that can cause excessive urination in men, which is especially annoying at night.

POSSIBLE BENEFITS

Good expectorant—clears chest of congestion.

Soothing to sexual organs.

May help relieve excessive urination due to benign enlarged prostate.

How to Use It

ORALLY

EXTRACT:
Mix 30 to 60 drops in liquid daily.

CAUTION

Any man who is experiencing pain or swelling of the prostate, or who is having difficulty with urination, or who passes any blood in the urine, should be examined by his physician.

SHIITAKE MUSHROOM

(*Lentinus edodes*)

FACTS

These mushrooms contain a polysaccharide called lentinan that has been shown to slow the growth of cancerous tumors in animals. Studies suggest that lentinan may work by enhancing the immune system's ability to fight against infection. This mushroom is used as a cancer-fighting agent in Japan and China. Shiitake also lowers cholesterol, which helps prevent heart disease.

POSSIBLE BENEFITS

Boosts the immune system.

Lowers blood cholesterol.

How to Use It

ORALLY

CAPSULES:
Take 1 up to 3 times daily.

CAUTION

Seek professional advice before using this or any other herb to treat cancer or tumors.

SKULLCAP

(Scutellaria lateriflora)

FACTS

As its name implies, the flower of this plant resembles a cap. This herb is known for its calming effect on the body. An antispasmodic, it has been used to relieve menstrual cramps and muscle pain due to stress. It is given to recovering alcoholics suffering from withdrawal symptoms. Also called "mad dog weed," skullcap is a traditional remedy for rabies. One old herbal recommends this herb for "explosive headaches of school teachers with frequent urination." Another claims that it soothes excessive sexual desires (this was written when this condition was considered a problem—long prior to the sexual revolution!).

POSSIBLE BENEFITS

Helps reduce nervous tension.

Good for insomnia.

Good for muscle tension.

How to Use It

ORALLY

CAPSULES:
Take 1 capsule up to 3 times daily.
DRIED HERB:
Mix 1 tablespoon herb with 8 ounces warm water.
Drink 1 cup of the tea daily.
EXTRACT:
Mix 3 to 12 drops in liquid daily.

SLIPPERY ELM BARK
(Ulmus fulva)

FACTS

There's a high level of mucilage in the bark of this tree, which makes it extremely soothing for scratchy, raw, sore throats and mouth irritations. It is also good for the sore feeling that often follows vomiting. Some herbalists also use it to relieve pain of gastric ulcers.

POSSIBLE BENEFITS

Provides soothing coating to throat and esophagus.

How to Use It

ORALLY

LOZENGES:
Take 1 up to 3 times daily.

SUMA

(*Pfaffia paniculata*)

FACTS

Dubbed "para todo" or "for all things," by Brazilian Indian tribes who first discovered the medicinal uses of this herb, suma is the South American version of ginseng. South of the border, it is used as a tonic. In North America, it has been used to treat exhaustion resulting from debilitating viral infections such as Epstein-Barr disease and the mysterious chronic fatigue syndrome.

WHAT IT CAN DO FOR YOU

Energy tonic.

Fights fatigue.

How to Use It

ORALLY

CAPSULES OR TABLETS:
Take 1 or 2 up to 3 times daily (for a total of 6).

PERSONAL ADVICE

This herb can help perk up people who are recovering from the flu, as well as anyone else who lacks energy and stamina.

TURMERIC
(Circuma longa)

FACTS

Turmeric is a spice that is a common ingredient in curry powder, usually in combination with other herbs such as cayenne, garlic, cumin, and onion. Due to its antibacterial properties, turmeric is believed to have been used to preserve food before the widespread use of refrigeration. More than three thousand years ago, Indian healers used turmeric to treat obesity. We now know that turmeric has a beneficial effect on the liver, stimulating the flow of bile and the breakdown of dietary fats. In Asia, turmeric was used to treat stomach disorders, menstrual problems, blood clots, and liver-related ailments such as jaundice. Modern research performed primarily in Germany and India shows that turmeric protects against gallbladder disease and can also be used as an effective treatment for it. Studies also confirm that this herb is useful for preventing blood clots. A potent antiinflammatory, herbalists recommend turmeric for the pain and swelling of arthritis.

POSSIBLE BENEFITS

Helps prevent sticking together of blood cells that could cause dangerous clots.

Good for liver function.

Helps prevent gallbladder disease.

Relieves symptoms of arthritis.

How to Use It

ORALLY

CAPSULES:
Take 1 (300-mg) capsule up to 3 times daily.

PERSONAL ADVICE

A delicious way to get more turmeric in your diet is to eat more curry. The herbs that are combined to make curry help prevent heart disease and stroke by reducing cholesterol and preventing blood clots.

UVA URSI

(Arctostaphylos uva ursi)

FACTS

Also known as bearberry, uva ursi's use as a folk remedy for urinary tract infections has been validated by modern research showing that this herb is an effective treatment for bladder and kidney ailments. Uva ursi is also an excellent diuretic.

POSSIBLE BENEFITS

Relieves pain from cystitis and nephritis.

Eliminates excessive bloating due to water retention.

How to Use It

ORALLY

CAPSULES:
Take 1 up to 3 times daily to relieve symptoms.
DRIED HERB:
Mix 1 tablespoon in 8 ounces warm water. Drink 1
cup daily.

VALERIAN

(*Valeriana officinalis*)

FACTS

Dubbed the "Valium of the nineteenth century," valerian
(chemically unrelated to Valium) is recognized worldwide
for its relaxing effect on the body. In Europe, it is often
prescribed to treat anxiety. Unlike many of the prescription drugs commonly used in the United States for this
purpose—such as Valium and Xanax—valerian has few
unpleasant side effects (other than the fact that it doesn't
taste very good) and it is not addictive. Valerian offers
another advantage over Valium. Valium has a synergistic
effect with alcohol: When taken together, the two drugs
greatly exaggerate each other's effect on the body. Not
only does this synergistic relationship encourage abuse
but when combined the two drugs can pose serious side
effects. For centuries, valerian has been the treatment of
choice by herbalists for nervous tension and panic attacks.
It also has been used to relieve muscle cramps related to
stress, menstrual cramps, and PMS. Although valerian has
been widely studied, how this herb works is still not
known.

POSSIBLE BENEFITS

Calms you down.

Relieves insomnia.

Good for muscle tension.

Good for periods of extreme emotional stress.

Relieves gas pains and stomach cramps.

How to Use It

ORALLY

CAPSULES:
   Take 1 up to 3 times daily to relieve symptoms.
EXTRACT:
   Mix 10 drops in liquid daily.

CAUTION

In extremely high dosages, valerian may cause paralysis and a weakening of the heartbeat. Therefore, do not exceed recommended dose.

WHITE WILLOW BARK

(*Salix alba*)

FACTS

For centuries, a derivative of this bark called salicum was used to break fevers, soothe headaches, and reduce pain and swelling in arthritic joints. Based on their studies of salicum, researchers derived a synthetic drug called acetyl salicylic acid—better known today as aspirin. Unlike aspirin, which can cause stomach irritation, white willow contains tannins, which are actually good for the digestive system.

POSSIBLE BENEFITS

Reduces inflammation.

Relieves pain.

Good for neuralgia.

Relieves swollen joints due to rheumatism and arthritis.

How to Use It

ORALLY

CAPSULES:
Take 2 every 2 to 3 hours as needed.

PERSONAL ADVICE

This is an excellent aspirin substitute.

YERBA SANTA
(Eriodictyon californicum)

FACTS

The American Indians smoked or chewed the leaves of this plant as a treatment for asthma. It is still used by herbal enthusiasts for bronchial congestion, asthma, and hayfever.

POSSIBLE BENEFITS

Quiets a nagging cough.

Helps clear chest of phlegm.

Relieves congestion due to allergy.

How to Use It

ORALLY

DRIED HERB:
  Mix 1 tablespoon of herb in 8 ounces warm water.
  Drink 1 cup daily.
EXTRACT:
  Mix 10 to 20 drops in liquid daily.

YUCCA
(Yucca liliaceae)

FACTS

The Southwestern Indians have used this herb for hundreds of years to treat pain and inflammation of arthritis and rheumatism.

POSSIBLE BENEFITS

Reduces inflammation.

Relieves joint pain due to arthritis and rheumatism.

How to Use It

ORALLY

CAPSULES OR TABLETS:
 Take 1 up to 3 times daily to relieve symptoms.
EXTRACT:
 Mix 10 to 30 drops in liquid up to 3 times daily.

CAUTION

Long-term use may slow the absorption of fat-soluble vitamins such as A, D, E, and K. Check with your health professional to see if supplements of these oil-soluble vitamins are needed if you are using yucca over a period of time.

UP-AND-COMING HERBS

Although these "up-and-coming" herbs have not quite achieved the status of the "Hot Hundred," they are growing in popularity in the United States and are beginning to attract a loyal following.

OSHA

(*Ligusticum porteri*)

FACTS

This herb was originally used by western Native Americans to treat colds, flu, and upper respiratory infections. Osha is purported to be an immune builder, that is, it helps the body ward off viral infections. It is now sold in combination with lomatuum root, another reputed immune enhancer used by Native Americans, in capsule form. As word gets out about Osha's positive action on the immune system, it will undoubtedly become as popular as echinacea, astragalus, and other well-known herbal immune boosters.

HOW TO USE IT

Take 1 capsule up to 3 times daily. Mix 20 to 30 drops of extract in liquid up to 3 times daily.

CHASTE TREE OR VITEX

(*Verbenaceae* species)

FACTS

Vitex (also known as chaste tree and agnus castus) is extremely popular in Europe where it is used to treat PMS as well as some of the unpleasant side effects associated with menopause. For centuries, this herb has been reputed to be a hormone balancer and was at one time recommended as a treatment for excessive sexual desire. European herbalists use it today to treat fibroid tumors and other female complaints. As the baby-boom generation passes into menopause, I believe that this herb will be rediscovered by women looking for a natural alternative to estrogen replacement therapy.

HOW TO USE IT

Take 1 capsule up to 3 times daily. Mix 10 to 30 drops of extract in liquid up to 3 times daily.

REISHI MUSHROOM

(*Ganoderma lucidum*)

FACTS

Recent studies show that extracts from this delicious mushroom, which is popular in Oriental cuisines, can stop the growth of cancerous tumors in mice. More research needs to be done to determine if it has the same effect on humans. Other studies have confirmed that this mushroom has a strong antihistamine action that can help control allergies. Similar to shiitake mushroom, reishi can lower cholesterol and help prevent blood clots.

HOW TO USE IT

Take 1 capsule up to 3 times daily.

HERBAL TEAS AND THEIR USES

There are two kinds of herbal teas: those that are used primarily as alternative beverages to coffee and regular tea, and those that are valued for their medicinal properties. The former are sold in supermarkets and the herbs are merely used as flavoring agents. These teas are relatively weak and generally harmless, but they do not offer the same benefits of real herbal tea. The real stuff is usually sold in health food stores and herb shops in tea bags or dried herbs. As a rule, these herbal preparations are more potent than the supermarket variety and should be used more carefully. Before you use any herbal tea, however, you should learn as much as possible about the herb. If you are pregnant or have a medical condition such as high blood pressure, check with your doctor before drinking any herbal tea. Avoid

---

using stimulants such as ephedra at night, or soporific (relaxing) herbs such as chamomile early in the day when you may need a lift. Some manufacturers may add caffeine to their packaged herbal products, so if you want to avoid this drug, be sure to read the label very carefully. Your best bet is to buy an herbal tea that is labeled "caffeine-free."

Making an herbal tea is about as simple as boiling water. Put 1 tablespoon of the herb in a tea ball and place in 1 cup of boiling water. Let the mixture simmer for five to ten minutes. Remove the tea ball and drink. If you don't want to use a tea ball, simply steep the herbs directly in the hot water and strain after ten minutes. To make several cups at once, use a glass or ceramic tea pot. Use 1 tablespoon of herb for every cup ofwater. You can sweeten your home-brewed tea with sugar or honey.

In warm weather, you can add ice cubes to the prepared tea to make your own iced tea. Peppermint, apple, chamomile, cranberry, raspberry, and orange flower are particularly good when chilled. Garnish with lemon or a sprig of fresh mint.

The following is a list of popular herbal teas and a brief description of their reputed uses.

Alfalfa tea—Aids digestion

Angelica tea—Mild antispasmodic and digestive aid

Aniseed tea—Decongestant for nose and sinuses

Basil and borage tea—"Pick-me-up" tonic

Bilberry tea—Aids circulation

Black currant tea—Stimulates taste buds

Blueberry tea—Pleasant before-meal tea

Borage tea—Antimelancholy

Buchu tea—Natural diuretic (dangerous if taken to excess)

Burdock root tea—Helps sciatica and rheumatoid arthritis

Butcher's broom—Good diuretic

Catnip tea—Relaxant and mild depressant

Chamomile tea—Calms hyperactive children; good before bedtime

Chicory tea—Normalizes liver function

Cinnamon tea—Clears the brain and improves throught processes

Cornsilk tea—Reduces pain of urinary infections

Couch grass tea—Tightens and tones up the bladder sphincter, good diuretic

Dandelion tea—Improves liver function and kidney function

Elder flowers tea—Increases immune function

Fennel tea—Good for the pancreas

Fenugreek tea—Good for colds, clogged ears, and aching sinuses

Ginger tea—Appetite restorer

Ginseng tea—Natural tonic for a "lift"

Goldenseal root tea—Internal detergent (avoid if you have high blood pressure)

Hawthorne berries tea—Energizing to the elderly

Hops tea—Relaxant and calming agent

Horehound tea—Helps loosen heavy mucus

Jasmine tea—Mild nerve sedative

Juniper berries tea—Helps cystitis or bladder inflammation

Licorice tea—Good laxative

Mate tea—Tones muscles, especially the smooth muscles of the heart

Nettle tea—Increases blood pressure (avoid if you have high blood pressure)

Orange flowers tea—Sleep aid

Parsley tea—Diuretic (increases flow of urine)

Peppermint tea—Antigas

Raspberry tea—Tightens, tones, and strengthens the uterus

Red clover tea—Inner cleanser

Rosehips tea—Adrenal stimulant during daytime

Sage tea—Improves brain nourishment; known as the "thinker's tea"

Sarsaparilla tea—Laxative, hormone balancer (should not be used on a regular basis)

Senna tea—Strong laxative

Slippery elm bark—Pain reliever

Spearmint tea—Antigas

Thyme tea—Sore throats and colds

Valerian tea—Natural sedative

Yarrow tea—General tonic

CHAPTER 3

Traditional Favorites

These time-honored herbs have been valued for centuries for their reputed medicinal properties. Although they may lack the cachet of the "Hot Hundred," they still have a strong following among traditional herbalists.

LEMON BALM

(Melissa officinalis)

FACTS

Originally grown in the Orient, Arab traders introduced this herb to Spain. It was later brought to Germany by Benedictine monks. Still popular in Europe, lemon balm is now grown in parts of the United States. A member of the mint family, lemon balm contains volatile oils that provide its pleasant, lemony scent. This herb has long been a folk remedy for gas and colic. The famous seventeenth-century herbalist Culpeper thought so highly of lemon balm that he wrote, "Let a syrup made with the juice of it and sugar . . . be kept in every gentle woman's house to relieve the weak stomachs and sick bodies of their poor and sickly neighbours." Herbalists still prescribe this herb for upset stomach, nervous tension, and insomnia. A mild diaphoretic, lemon balm induces sweating when taken hot. This cools the body and can help break a fever.

HOW IT'S USED TODAY

This herb is widely available in tea, dried herb, and extract. Mix ½ to 1 teaspoon of extract in liquid up to 3 times daily. Use the dried herb to make tea, or drink 1 cup of packaged tea daily.

BORAGE
(Borago officinalis)

FACTS

In medieval times, borage tea was given to competitors in tournaments as a moral booster. "I, borage bring always courage," was a popular rhyme of the day. Culpeper noted that this herb can "increase milk in women's breasts," and was excellent for clearing phlegm from the lungs. Through the years, herbalists have used borage to treat a wide range of ailments, from ulcers to frazzled nerves. Borage is also an excellent source of gamma linoleic acid, which is used to treat symptoms of PMS.

HOW IT'S USED TODAY

This herb is available in extract and capsules. Take up to 3 capsules daily. Mix 1 teaspoon of extract in juice. Drink daily.

CARDAMOM

(Elletaria cardamonum)

FACTS

Grown in India, these pungent, aromatic seeds contain a large amount of volatile oil that helps stimulate digestion and relieve gas. A mild stimulant, cardamom is a standard ingredient in curry.

HOW IT'S USED TODAY

For indigestion, mix 15 pulverized seeds in ½ cup hot water. Add 1 ounce of fresh gingerroot and a cinnamon stick. Simmer 15 minutes over low heat. Add ½ cup milk and simmer 10 more minutes. Add 2 to 3 drops of vanilla. Sweeten with honey. Drink 1 to 2 cups daily.

CHICKWEED

(Stellaria media)

FACTS

Culpeper wrote that chickweed "boiled with hog's grease applied, helpeth cramps, convulsions and palsy." In folk medicine, this herb has been used as an expectorant and an antacid. Used externally in ointment form, is it reputed to be excellent for bruises, irritations, eczema, and other skin problems.

HOW IT'S USED TODAY

Take 1 capsule up to 3 times daily. Use ointment as needed.

CLUB MOSS

(*Lycopodium clavatum*)

FACTS

American Indians used to sprinkle a powder made from this herb on wounds to stop bleeding. It was also an old-time treatment for rheumatism.

HOW IT'S USED TODAY

The powder is sold in health food stores and herb shops. Use on minor skin wounds.

CUCUMBER

(*Cucumis sativus*)

FACTS

Since ancient times, the juice of the cucumber has been used as a facial cleanser and as a treatment for skin irritations. Cleopatra herself was reputed to have used cucumber to preserve her beautiful skin. Culpeper recommends cucumber for sunburns and freckles. Eaten as a vegetable, cucumber is a good diuretic and can help prevent constipation. Researchers are now investigating an extract of cucumber as a possible "cholesterol buster."

HOW IT'S USED TODAY

Place cucumber slices on irritated areas. Eat the fresh vegetable. Cucumber juice is also used in many skin products.

ELECAMPANE

(*Inula helenium*)

FACTS

This herb is a traditional remedy for respiratory tract infections and digestive problems. It is not only a good expectorant but its essential oils and high mucilage content provide a soothing, protective coating that can relieve irritation due to excessive coughing. Culpeper endorsed elecampane wholeheartedly: "It has not its equal in the cure of whooping-cough in children, when all other medicines fail." Once held in high regard by the medical establishment, this herb was listed in the *U.S. Pharmacopeia*. Elecampane was also a folk cure for amenorrhea, or loss of menstruation. (This or any other herb that can induce menstruation should not be used during pregnancy.)

HOW IT'S USED TODAY

Use the dried herb to make tea. Drink 1 cup daily. Mix 10 to 30 drops of extract in liquid. Drink up to 3 times daily.

ICELAND MOSS

(*Centraria islandica*)

FACTS

This plant is not a moss at all, but a plant form called a lichen, which is made up of a fungus and alga. Still used to treat tuberculosis in some parts of the world, iceland moss is a folk remedy for coughs and congestion due to colds.

HOW IT'S USED TODAY

Use the dried herb to make tea. Mix 1 teaspoon of the herb in ½ cup hot water daily. For best results, sip slowly. Use this herb only to treat specific symptoms. Do not use it for more than two weeks at a time.

LAVENDER
(*Lavendula officinalis*)

FACTS

This member of the mint family has an extremely popular scent that is used in perfumes, soaps, and sachets. The early Romans used lavender to scent their public baths; the herb's name is derived from the Latin word *lavare*, which means to wash. In aromatherapy, lavender oil is used to promote relaxation and treat headaches. Lavender tea is a traditional remedy for "gassy stomach," and for relieving anxiety.

HOW IT'S USED TODAY

Mix 5 drops of essential oil in warm water for a soothing bath.

MEADOWSWEET
(*Filipendula ulmaria*)

FACTS

This herb was reputed to be the favorite of Queen Elizabeth I because of its sweet, fragrant scent. Long a remedy for flu, fever, and arthritis, meadowsweet contains an aspirin-type compound called salicylic acid. The tea is regarded as an excellent diuretic.

HOW IT'S USED TODAY

Make tea from the dried herb. Drink 1 cup daily.

MOTHERWORT

(*Leonurus cardiaca*)

FACTS

Since ancient times, this herb has been used to treat "female problems" and as a cardiotonic. The Greeks used motherwort to relieve the pain from childbirth and as a tranquilizer. Culpeper wrote, "There is no better herb to take melancholy vapours from the heart and to strengthen it." Modern herbalists used motherwort to treat PMS. In combination with other "women's herbs" such as raspberry leaves, it is believed to help prepare the uterus for delivery and labor.

HOW IT'S USED TODAY

Mix 10 to 15 drops of extract in warm liquid up to 3 times daily. Use dried herb to make tea. Drink 1 cup daily.

CAUTION

Do not use during pregnancy.

MUSTARD (WHITE AND BLACK)

(Brassica hirta)
(Brassica nigra)

FACTS

Both varieties of mustard plant have similar properties, although black mustard is regarded as the stronger of the two. Culpeper recommended that mustard be used externally for joint pain and sciatica (backache) and be taken internally with honey for coughs. Through the years, herbalists have pretty much followed his advice. Today, however, mustard is usually used externally.

HOW IT'S USED TODAY

Mustard oil diluted with rubbing alcohol can be applied to the skin to increase the flow of blood to arthritic areas. Never use the undiluted oil; it can be very irritating. When I was a child, my mother used to apply a mustard plaster to my chest when I had a bad cold—the warming action of the mustard was very soothing. The plaster is easy to make with prepared mustard powder. Mix cold water with the powder to make a thick paste. Spread the paste on a clean cloth and put a layer of gauze over the mustard. Apply to the chest or to arthritic joints. Remove after 10 minutes. Prolonged use can result in skin irritation. The leaves of the white mustard plant can be used in salad and are quite tasty.

ROSEMARY

(Rosmarinus officinalis)

FACTS

Culpeper wrote that this herb was good for "diseases of the head and brain, as the giddiness and swimming therein." Herbalists still use rosemary to treat dizziness due to inner ear disturbances. Through the years, rosemary has been touted as the herb that can sharpen the memory. When rubbed on the temples, the essential oil can provide great relief from headaches, especially migraines. Mixed with olive oil, a few drops of rosemary oil or leaves are a popular hair treatment for dandruff and are believed by herbalists to stimulate hair growth. Sipped as a tea, this herb is reputed to be good for nervous tension and is especially good if you have tension headaches and you want to reach for something natural. Rosemary is also a very popular cooking herb.

HOW IT'S USED TODAY

The oil is used for aromatherapy (see page 265). Make a tea from the dried herb. Drink daily.

HAMLET ON HERBS

Rosemary is an ancient folk remedy for improving memory. Wrote Shakespeare in Hamlet, "That's Rosemary, that's for remembrance; I pray you, love, remember."

SAGE
(*Salvia officinalis*)

FACTS

This herb's botanical name is derived from the Latin *salvere*, which means to save, a testimony to sage's early reputation as a cure-all. In the Middle Ages, sage was used to prevent the night sweats typical of tuberculosis patients. Herbalists still recommend it for people who suffer from excessive perspiration. Culpeper prescribed sage tea as a mouthwash for sore gums. The tea is also used for stomach cramps and gas. A popular cooking herb, sage is reputed to be good for the digestion.

HOW IT'S USED TODAY

Make a tea from the dried herb. Drink daily. Use tea as a gargle for sore gums up to 3 times daily. Use this delicious herb in your cooking.

THYME
(*Thymus vulgaris*)

FACTS

In the Middle Ages, thyme was believed to increase courage: Women would give a sprig of thyme to their favorite knights before they went into battle. Culpeper wrote that thyme was "a strengthener of the lungs," and "taken internally, comforts the stomach much, and expels wind." Through the years, thyme has been used as an expectorant and a disinfectant and is known for its antifungal properties. It also makes a good gargle for sore throats.

HOW IT'S USED TODAY

Make a tea from the dried herb. Drink daily, or gargle with it up to 3 times daily. Rub extract between toes for athlete's foot daily. The extract can also be applied externally for crabs, lice, and scabies. Use daily.

WILD OREGON GRAPE

(*Mahonia aquifolium*)

FACTS

Native to North America, this herb became popular in Europe as a "blood purifier." Wild oregon grape is believed to enhance liver function and is used to treat jaundice, hepatitis, and other liver ailments. It is also reputed to be good for eczema and psoriasis. This herb is also used as a diuretic. It is widely available in extract and dried herb.

HOW IT'S USED TODAY

Make tea from dried herb. Drink daily. Mix 10 to 30 drops of extract in liquid daily.

WITCH HAZEL

(*Hamamelis virginiana*)

FACTS

First used by North American Indians, witch hazel is an essential item for every home medicine cabinet. Available in liquid extract, witch hazel's antiinflammatory action is very soothing for minor scrapes, cuts, and bruises. Applied directly to hemorrhoids and varicose veins, it helps relieve the pain and inflammation typical of these conditions. Splashed on the face, it is a revitalizing skin tonic that helps eliminate excess oil.

HOW IT'S USED TODAY

Apply factory-distilled extract to irritated areas several times daily.

HERBS IN THE BIBLE

On the third day of creation God said, "Let the earth bring forth grass, the herb yielding seed, and the fruit tree yielding fruit after his kind, whose seed is in itself upon the earth: and it was so."

—Genesis

Throughout the Old and New Testaments—from the Garden of Eden through the Gospels—there are numerous references to herbs that were commonly used in biblical times. The Fertile Crescent, one of the earliest centers of civilization, was full of orchards, woods, and lush, tropical vegetation. The first man, Adam, was a gardener and his son, Cain, grew vegetables. Our ancestors literally lived off the land, and as a result, had a great respect for nature. The ancient Hebrews believed that nature was a gift from God and held His creation in very high esteem.

Herbs such as cinnamon, pomegranate bark, aloe, garlic, onions, cloves, and saffron are frequently mentioned throughout the Bible. On at least one occasion, an herb actually plays an important role in the story line. In Genesis, Leah and Rachel, both wives of Jacob, were constantly vying for his favor. Leah had conceived many sons for Jacob, but Rachel had remained barren. When Leah's son Reuben finds a mandrake, a reputed aphrodisiac, Rachel pleads with Leah to give it to her. In exchange for the precious fruit, Rachel agrees to let Leah spend the night with Jacob. Leah promptly conceives another child, but later, so does Rachel. To this day, mandrakes are called "love apples" in the Middle East, and are still valued for their supposed aphrodisiac qualities.

The Ancient Hebrews apparently had a healthy reverence for plant medicines. In Ecclesiastes, we are told, "The Lord created medicines from the earth, and a sensible man doesn't despise them."

The Bible also forbids short-term exploitation of the land, a rule that future generations have chosen to ignore. For example, in Leviticus, there are many laws concerning the preservation of trees. God says, "Thou shalt not destroy the trees thereof by forcing an axe against them: for thou may eatest of them, and thou shalt not cut them down (for the tree of the field is man's life)."

CHAPTER 4

Herbs from Around the World

Nearly every culture has developed its own style of herbal medicine. Although many rely on the same herbs, each nationality has left its own unique imprint on this universal healing system. In this chapter, I focus on four different forms of herbal healing that I feel have greatly influenced the practice of herbal medicine today: the Chinese system, the Ayurvedic form of traditional medicine in India, Native American medicine, and South American medicine. *Note*: Herbs that are also included in the "Hot Hundred" are designated by an asterisk*. See "Hot Hundred" entries for more information.

CHINESE HERBAL TRADITION

Since the resumption of U.S. diplomatic relations with China in the 1970s, Westerners have been exposed to China's rich tradition of healing that dates back more than four thousand years. The first known Chinese medical book, the *Wu Shi Er Bing Fang* (*Prescriptions for Fifty-two Diseases*), was compiled around three thousand years ago. It includes 283 prescriptions for fifty-two diseases including malaria, skin ulcers, and warts. The *Shen Nong Ben Cao Jing*, China's first bona-fide herbal, is about two thousand years old. It includes more than five hundred plants used for their medicinal purposes. The plant drugs were divided into three categories. The first group, the superior drugs, were herbs that were considered to be nontoxic and therefore were safe for daily consumption as tonics. The second group, the so-called medium drugs, were not considered entirely benign and could be toxic under certain circumstances. The third group, the inferior drugs, were classified as toxic and were only used on a short-term basis to treat specific problems, much the same way we use potent antibiotics today. Many of the herbs listed in the *Shen Nong* herbal are still used today in a similar fashion by Chinese physicians.

The modern Chinese use some five thousand plants and animal substances as healing agents. To date, only a handful of these remedies have been seriously investigated.

Traditionally, the Chinese approach to medicine has differed sharply from that of the West. Unlike Western medicine, the emphasis in China is not to eradicate disease but to promote health. For example, in China, many herbs are taken as tonics, that is, they are used to enhance physical and mental well-being, not to treat a specific illness. However, in Western medicine, there are no tonics. Drugs are prescribed only for the sick.

Another major difference is that in the West, medicine is considered pure science. This is not so in the Orient. Chinese medicine is an interesting blend of philosophy and healing. The goal of the healer is to restore balance and harmony to the body. The philosophy behind traditional Chinese medicine is very complex, and it is impossible to do it justice in a few paragraphs. However, the "law of yin and yang"—known as "The Great Principle" to the Chinese—can shed some light on the Chinese outlook. The Chinese believe that nature is divided into two opposing cycles: yin and yang. Yang represents an action or activity that expends energy. Yin represents a more contemplative, restful phase in which energy is replenished. The Chinese believe that maintaining a proper balance of yin and yang is essential to maintaining good health. In Western terms, Chinese medicine takes a "holistic" approach to healing: Health is defined in both spiritual and physical terms.

In the West, we are just beginning to explore the relationship between body and mind, and in that respect, we are light-years behind the Chinese. In recent years, we have begun to take a serious look at Chinese medicine, which may yield some promising results in terms of new drugs and therapies.

The following list describes the thirty-one most popular Chinese herbs that are available in the United States. Some are so popular that they are cited in the "Hot Hundred." For information on how to use them, refer to the "Hot Hundred" listing. Although many of the better-known Chinese herbs are available at health food stores and herb shops, some of the more exotic ones are only available in oriental herb shops, which are generally found in urban Chinatowns. Using these herbs may require special preparation; therefore, if you want to try one of the more exotic herbs, you should consult with a Chinese herbal practitioner.

Some of the herbs listed in this section have more than one Chinese name due to variations in dialect. Not all of the herbs are familiar to Westerners or have English names.

191

Top Thirty Chinese Herbs

MUXU OR ZIMU
(Western name: Alfalfa*)

FACTS

The first documented use of this herb by the Chinese dates back to the sixth century. Chinese healers use alfalfa to treat kidney stones and to relieve fluid retention and swelling.

BA DAN XING REN
(Western name: Almond*)

FACTS

As far back as 200 B.C., the Chinese have used almond oil as a local anesthetic and muscle relaxer.

LU HUI
(Western name: Aloe vera*)

FACTS

Aloe has been used for at least two thousand years by the Chinese. It was taken internally as a laxative, and to promote healing of disorders of the stomach, liver, and spleen. Externally, the gel was used to treat burns. Today, the Chinese have used aloe gel against radiation and thermal burns, chapped and dry skin, leg ulcers, and skin disorders.

LUOLE

(Western name: Basil*)

FACTS

Since the sixth century, basil has been used to improve blood circulation and to enhance the digestion. Externally, it is used to soothe bloodshot eyes and relieve itching from hives.

DOU FU-TOFU

(Western name: Bean curd)

FACTS

Since 200 B.C., tofu has been cooked into a soup to treat colds—the Chinese version of chicken soup. Externally, it has been used to promote healing of ulcers and sores. Sold in many greengrocers, tofu is becoming popular as a meat substitute. Tofu can be stored up to five days in the refrigerator. To preserve freshness, immerse tofu in water and change water daily. Tofu is usually added raw to hot soup, and can be sautéed in a wok with other vegetables. It is both low in calories and highly nutritious: A six-ounce portion is a mere 100 calories and contains about 6 percent protein.

YE JU

(Western name: Chrysanthemum)

FACTS

A homemade "tea" made from this flower is used to treat conjunctivitis and skin diseases. Taken internally, it is reputed to lower blood pressure.

> **TO LIFE!**
>
> In China, dried chrysanthemum flowers are a symbol of longevity. They are floated in a cup of tea served to guests as a way of wishing them a long life.

PU GONG YING

(Western name: Dandelion*)

FACTS

Since the seventh century, the Chinese have known about the antibacterial properties of the juice of this flower. Dandelion tea is a popular treatment for upper respiratory infections and is sold in many health food stores and herb shops. Drink 1 cup daily.

HU SUAN

(Western name: Garlic*)

FACTS

Since the early sixth century, the Chinese have used garlic as an antibiotic and an antiinflammatory. It is still an extremely popular herb in China, and is used to treat amebic dysentery, yeast infections, and middle ear infections. Externally, it is used for nosebleeds and snake and insect bites.

GAN JIANG

(Western name: Ginger*)

FACTS

For two thousand years, the Chinese have used this herb to treat nausea, vomiting, and motion sickness. It is still one of the best remedies available for these kinds of problems. You can buy the fresh root in the produce section at most grocery stores. Commercial preparations are sold in health food stores.

REN SHEN

(Western name: Ginseng*)

FACTS

Books have been written about this amazing herb, known as the "King of Tonics." The Chinese revere ginseng. A Chinese herbalist from 200 B.C. said it best when he wrote that ginseng can "vitalize the five organs, calm the nerves, stop palpitations due to fright, brighten vision, increase intellect and with long-term use, prolong life and make one feel young."

GAN CAO

(Western name: Licorice*)

FACTS

The Chinese have used this herb for more than five thousand years! It reduces fever and inflammation, promotes healing of wounds, and is good for sore throats and coughs. Licorice stimulates the production of bile by the liver and can relieve stomachaches and ulcers. We now know that this herb also lowers cholesterol.

FAN MU GUA

(Western name: Papaya*)

FACTS

This herb is a sixteenth-century remedy for indigestion and constipation. To date, it is still one of the best.

FAN JIA

(Western name: Hot pepper)

FACTS

An excellent source of vitamin C, the biting hot peppers typical of some Chinese cuisine have been used as a digestive aid and appetite stimulant.

MI DIE XIANG

(Western name: Rosemary)

FACTS

Since the third century, the Chinese have used this fragrant herb to treat headaches and stomachaches. It is also believed to have a calming effect on the nervous system.

HUANG CHI
(Western name: Astragalus)*

FACTS

This is a current favorite among the Chinese, especially those who are physically active. It is used as a tonic to improve the body's resistance to disease and is considered an energizer. Astragalus is also a diuretic and a digestive aid. This herb can be found in most health food stores and herb shops.

BUPLERUM OR CH'AI HU

FACTS

This herb is used to bring down a fever and relieve pain. It is also believed to reduce anxiety and helps relieve nausea.

LU RONG
(Western name: Deer antler)

FACTS

Since ancient times, the antler shed annually by deer were collected by healers and used in various forms as tonics. Deer antler is reputed to contain male hormones, which could explain its reputation as an aphrodisiac. Lu rong is used in many Chinese herbal preparations and is sold in capsule and extract form in Chinese herb shops and some health food stores. Follow directions on the package.

DONG QUAI* OR TANG KUEI

FACTS

This herb is highly valued in the Orient, and although it is called the "female ginseng," it is believed to be good for both sexes. For centuries, Chinese women have used this herb to treat gynecological problems such as menstrual cramps and PMS. Dong quai lowers blood pressure in both men and women, and is used as a treatment for insomnia. It should never be used during pregnancy. Dong quai is available in most health food stores and herb shops.

DON SEN OR TANG SHEN

FACTS

This herb is considered a milder version of ginseng and is used as a tonic and an energizer. Don Shen is also good for digestion and heartburn. This herb is sold in Chinese herb shops.

MA HUANG

(Western name: Ephedra*)

FACTS

The Chinese have traditionally used this herb to treat asthma. Today, compounds derived from this herb are commonly found in many over-the-counter cold and allergy medications. Ephedra is also a long-acting stimulant and should not be used by people with high blood pressure. American ephedra, known as Mormon tea or desert tea, is much milder than the Chinese variety and is used in a similar fashion. Ma huang is used in many natural cold remedies.

HO SHOU OR FO-TI

FACTS

Ho shou wu is known in China as a longevity herb. The Chinese believe that it is a rejuvenating tonic that can help preserve youthful vigor and energy. It is also believed to prevent gray hair and promote fertility in both sexes. Chinese studies show that extracts of this herb have antitumor properties. Ho shou wu is believed to prevent blood clots, lower blood pressure, and strengthen the heart. This herb is widely available in capsule and extract form in health food stores and herb shops.

DA T'SAO

(Western name: Jujube date)

FACTS

This herb has a calming effect on the body, and is used to treat insomnia and dizziness. Jujube is sold in Chinese herb shops.

GAY GEE

(Western name: Lycii)

FACTS

This herb is believed to increase longevity and promote cheerfulness. Chinese physicians use it as a treatment for high blood pressure, kidney disease, and some forms of cancer. Lycii can be found in most Chinese herb shops.

PAI SHU

FACTS

This herb is known for its diuretic properties and can be found in many Chinese herb shops.

PLATYCODON OR JIE ENG

FACTS

This herb is used to treat respiratory problems such as asthma, coughs, and bronchitis. It is also used for sore throats and lung ailments. Platycodon can be found at most Chinese herb shops.

PUERARIA OR KO KEN

FACTS

Chinese healers use this herb to treat colds, flu, and gastrointestinal problems. It can be purchased in Chinatown.

REHMANNIA OR SOK-DAY-SANG-DAY

FACTS

This herb is used to treat anemia, fatigue, and to promote the healing of injured bones. It is sold in Chinese herb shops.

SALVIA OR DANG SHEN

FACTS

Chinese women use this herb to promote menstrual regularity. It is sold in Chinese herb shops.

SCHIZANDRA FRUCTUS OR SCHIZANDRA CHINENSIS

FACTS

This herb is highly prized by Chinese women as a sexual enhancer and youth tonic. It is believed to preserve beauty and is a mild sedative. Schizandra is also reputed to increase sexual stamina among men. Until recently, this herb was rare and relatively expensive. It was highly coveted by the wealthy and a favorite among the Chinese emperors. Schizandra is also considered an adaptogen, and similar to ginseng, it is believed to increase stamina and fight against fatigue. It is also being touted as an antidepressant. Recent research supports some of these claims. According to a 1989 article in *Phytotherapy Research*, polo horses given schizandra performed better and showed better physiological responses to stress after taking the herb. Today, schizandra is widely available at health food stores and herb shops in capsules and extract. Follow directions on the package.

SILERIS OR FANG-FENG

FACTS

This herb is used to treat muscle spasms and is reputed to bolster the immune system. It can be found at most Chinese herb shops.

AN OLD REMEDY FOR AN OLD PROBLEM

In 1983, public health officials in Beijing, China, announced that a four-hundred-year-old prescription for treating hemorrhoids had been tested on 40,000 patients and proved to be 96 percent effective. The remedy: the injection of insect secretions on sumac leaves combined with crystal salts.

SOUTH AMERICAN HERBS

Ever since the first European explorers set foot in the New World, South America has been a fertile ground for plant medicines. To this day, much of the South American population still relies on herbal remedies. In urban centers in the United States with large Hispanic communities, the neighborhood botanica or herb shop often does a brisker business than the local pharmacy. Many herbs commonly used in the United States originated in South America; however, there are scores of others that have not yet found their way here. The following is a list of the hottest South American herbs. Some are already household names; the others, I predict, are destined to become them. Although this list includes some "Hot Hundred" herbs that are widely available in packaged form, some of the more obscure herbs may be sold in their natural state and require preparation. Be sure to check with a knowledgeable herbal practitioner before using an unfamiliar herb.

CAYENNE*
(Capsicum anuun or *Capsicum frutescens)*

FACTS

Native to northeastern coastal areas of South America, these red hot peppers have been used in folk medicine since 7000 B.C.!

GUARANA
(Paulina cupana)

FACTS

The seeds of this plant contain up to 5 percent caffeine and are well known for their stimulating effect. Guarana is reputed to increase mental alertness and fight fatigue. In Brazil, guarana is used in soft drinks. It is available in the United States in capsule form by itself or in combination with other herbs. Follow directions on the package or consult an herbal practitioner.

IPECAC
(Cephaelis ipecacuanha)

FACTS

Found in southwestern Brazil, this herb induces vomiting and therefore is a popular remedy for food poisoning and other kinds of poisoning. Syrup of ipecac is approved by the FDA and is sold in drugstores. The herb itself is very toxic except when diluted in syrup form. Because it induces vomiting, ipecac is often abused by teenage girls suffering from bulimia, an eating disorder characterized by gorging and purging. Although this herb is an essential for every household, doctors recommend that you do not keep it within the reach of teenagers who may be tempted to use it to lose weight.

CAUTION

It is not always appropriate to induce vomiting in cases of poisoning. Check with your physician or local poison alert hotline before giving this or any other drug to a poison victim.

MATE

(Ilex paraguarienesis)

FACTS

Once used as a folk remedy against scurvy, a beverage made out of the leaf of this plant is the national drink of Argentina. Mate contains caffeine as well as vitamins C, A, and B complex. In Argentina, mate is touted as an energizer and a tonic. In fact, it is so popular that the average Argentinian consumes about 11 pounds of mate annually.

MURIA PUAMA

(Ptychopetalum olacoides)

FACTS

The bark and roots of this plant are highly regarded by the Brazilians as a stimulant, stomach tonic, and treatment for rheumatism. This herb is reputed to be an aphrodisiac. Although muria puama is very popular in Brazil, it is not commonly used in the United States.

PAU D'ARCO*
(*Tabebuia* species)

FACTS

Also known as *Taheebo*, *Lapacho*, and *Ipe roxo*, this herb is a folk remedy in Brazil for cancer and fungal infections. Studies show that this herb indeed has antitumor and antifungal properties. Pau d'arco is widely available in the United States in capsules and extract form.

SARSAPARILLA*
(*Smilax officinalis*)

FACTS

Native to Central America, at the turn of the century, this herb was a popular flavor in root beers and soft drinks. It is currently used in the United States by bodybuilders as a nonsteroidal method of increasing muscle mass and is also touted as an aphrodisiac. However, chemical analysis has not found any evidence of testosterone or other male hormones in this herb.

STEVIA
(Stevia rebaudiana)

FACTS

Originally from Paraguay, this herb is two hundred times sweeter than sugar. It is used in Japan as a noncaloric sweetener, but has not been approved for this use in the United States. Dried stevia leaves are available at herb shops and botanicas and can be used in cooking instead of sugar.

SUMA*
(Pfaffia paniculata)

FACTS

This herb is an extremely popular tonic in Brazil, and is also used by women there to relieve the symptoms associated with menopause. As the baby-boom generation reaches menopause within the next decade, I predict that this herb, along with others that are reputed to ease the transition to menopause, will increase in popularity in the United States.

WILD MEXICAN YAM
(Diosorea mexicanan and Diosorea composita)

FACTS

Used by native women for birth control and to prevent miscarriage, this yam produces chemicals from which oral contraceptives and sex hormones are synthesized. Some women herbalists in the United States use an extract from this herb as a contraceptive. I do not advise using this or any other herb to prevent conception unless it is under the supervision of a qualified practitioner.

AYURVEDA: THE TRADITIONAL MEDICINE OF INDIA

More than five thousand years old, the traditional herbal medicine of India may be the oldest healing system in the world. Ayurveda is the combination of two Sanskrit words: *ayu*, which means life, and *veda*, which means knowledge. According to Indian folklore, this precious knowledge was passed down from the Creator, known as Brahma. Similar to the ancient Roman and Greek theories of medicine, Ayurveda classified herbs according to five elements: earth, water, fire, air, and ether. Herbs also were subdivided according to five tastes: sweet, sour, salty, pungent, bitter, and astringent. Similar to Chinese herbal tradition, Ayurveda emphasizes the prevention of disease through the pursuit of physical, mental, and spiritual health. In many ways, Ayurveda was way ahead of its time: It places as much importance on diet and lifestyle as it does on medicinal cures, a philosophy that twentieth-century physicians are finally beginning to accept.

Ayurveda is still widely practiced in India today. The message of Ayurveda is a simple one and best summed up by the following Indian saying: "May everyone be happy. May everyone be healthy. May everyone be holy. May there never be disharmony of any kind, anywhere."

Herbs used in Ayurveda include many of the same herbs that are popular in the West, including alfalfa, aloe vera, devil's claw, echinacea, goldenseal, licorice root, fennel, fenugreek, and turmeric, all "Hot Hundred" herbs.

SAVING A TREASURE

Within the past few decades, we have witnessed the destruction of half of the world's tropical rainforests. Every second, another 1.5 acres of rainforest disappears—adding up to 50 million acres per year. If present trends continue, by the first quarter of the twenty-first century, the tropical rainforest will become as extinct as the dinosaur. As more and more of this precious land is plundered by developers for its minerals and lumber, countless species of plants and animals are also doomed to extinction.

Unfortunately, we are decimating the plant life faster than we can study it. Less than 1 percent of all tropical rainforest plants have been adequately researched for their medicinal properties. This is especially tragic in light of the fact that 25 percent of all Western medicines are derived from rainforest plants. A whopping 70 percent of the three thousand plant species known for their anticancer properties originated in the rainforest. Tropical plants such as the rosy periwinkle have given us two of our most powerful weapons against cancer— vincristine and vinblastine. The Pilocarpus tree, native to South America, spawned a highly effective treatment for glaucoma.

Many of these "wonder drugs" were brought to our attention by the local medicine men or shamans, the main healthcare providers in these remote areas. As the rainforests are flattened by bulldozers, the secrets of the shamans will be lost forever along with numerous plant cures that could have saved countless numbers of lives.

For more information on preserving what's left of this precious resource, write: Rainforest Alliance, 270 Lafayette Street, Suite 512, New York, New York 10012.

Ayurveda also includes some exotic herbs that are just being discovered by the West. The following is a list of commonly used Ayurvedic herbs. Since these herbs have not been well researched in the West, I would not recommend using them unless it is under the supervision of a knowledgeable practitioner.

Popular Ayurvedic Herbs

AMALAKI
(Phyllanthus emblica)

FACTS

For thousands of years, this herb has been used to treat coughs, eating disorders, and to normalize bowel function. It is also used to treat skin diseases and tumors.

ASHWAGANDHA
(Withania somniforal)

FACTS

This herb is used to promote the healing of broken bones. It has a calming effect on the body.

BRAHMI
(Hydrocotyle asiatica)

FACTS

Brahmi is used to relieve anxiety and is also a treatment for epilepsy and leprosy.

GUDUCHI

(Tinosphora cordifolia)

FACTS

A traditional remedy for diabetes and ulcers. (This is considered to be strong medicine and should not be used without supervision.)

SHANKA PUSPI

(Convolvulus mycrophyllus)

FACTS

This herb is used to treat anxiety. It is also a mild painkiller.

VACHA

(Acorus calamus)

FACTS

This herb has a calming effect on the body. It is also reputed to be an aphrodisiac.

NATIVE AMERICAN HERBS

When the early settlers arrived in the United States there were more than two thousand tribes of Native Americans. Each tribe had its own system of herbal medicine that was in many ways far superior to the European style of healthcare practiced by the pioneers. In fact, the early settlers were startled to see Indians recovering from injuries that they considered to be fatal. Noted one observer, "I have seen many who have received four or five bullet or arrow wounds through the stomach and who are so perfectly cured of them that they do not suffer any inconvenience. Through the knowledge of simples [herbs] which they received from their fathers, they will cure hands, arms and feet that our best surgeons would not hesitate to cut."

The typical tribal medicine man was as well equipped as any modern pharmacy to treat a wide range of medical needs, ranging from the common cold to birth control. Although we have incorporated some Native American herbs into our herbal tradition—in fact, some have even made it into the "Hot Hundred"—many have been forgotten or are difficult to obtain. Although you will not be able to locate most of these herbs at the local health food store, I have included a list of Native American herbal remedies for common problems to show how sophisticated this so-called primitive culture really was.

COLDS

Wungobe—Balsam fir

Nakadonup—Wild buckwheat

Ya-Tombe—Creosote bush

Aqui he binga—Blue gilia

Toza—Indian balsam

Taba emul—Meadow rye

Toya bawana—Horsemint

Batipi—Wild peony

SORE THROAT

Ax six sixie—Bitterroot

Pakitoki—Double bladder pod

Quit chemboo—Licorice root*

Pooy sonib—String plant

A sat chiot sake—Rattle weed

EYE PROBLEMS

Apos-ipoco—Alum root

So yaits—Pink plumes

Pah oh pimb—Acacia or cat claw

Sebu mogoonobu—Back turtle

KIDNEY AND BLADDER AILMENTS

Poku erop—Iris flag

Kube—Sage, bud

Sammapo—Juniper berries*

LAXATIVES

Bossowey—Sweet anise*

Ae buchoko—Cascara sagrada*

Kosi tsube—Gray willow

RHEUMATISM

Wapi—Juniper*

Pennikinni—Wormwood

Yano—Wild rose

TOOTHACHE

Poku erop—Iris

Pannonzia—Yarrow

Segumogoonbu—Nettleback

BIRTH CONTROL

Notmisha—Stoneseed

Sammapo—Juniper berries*

CHEWING GUM

Wahanane—Desert gum plant

SHAMPOO

Datil or viemp—Yucca*

Amole Indian—Soap root

If there were no plants, we wouldn't be here. We breathe in what they breathe out. That is how we learn from them.

—Keetwuah, a well-known Cherokee healer

CHAPTER 5

The Herbal Medicine Cabinet

Centuries before our medicine cabinets were jammed with over-the-counter medicines, our ancestors were treating themselves and their families with healing agents derived from the plant kingdom. There was an herbal remedy for just about every malady known to man, woman, and child—from fever to fatigue—and many worked surprisingly well. In this chapter, I have compiled a list of some home remedies that I feel still belong in the modern medicine cabinet. Do not give any herbs to children without first consulting with your pediatrician. *Note*: Herbs listed in the "Hot Hundred" are designated by an asterisk (*). See the "Hot Hundred" entries for more information.

THE BEST HERBS FOR COLDS, COUGHS, AND FLU

Ephedra* (ma huang) tea or cold preparations relieve congestion. (Ephedra is a long-acting stimulant and should not be used at night or by people who have high blood pressure. Avoid during pregnancy.) Follow directions on package.

Use 1 to 5 drops of eucalyptus* oil in a vaporizer to produce a soothing steam that helps clear clogged nasal passages.

Cayenne* tea reduces the discomfort caused by colds and helps warm the body. Take this one for chills! Cayenne is available in dried herb and prepared teas. For tea, use 1 teaspoon of dried herb in 1 cup hot water.

Fenugreek* tea is a good expectorant and is also soothing for sore throats. Fenugreek is available in dried herb and extract. For tea, use 1 teaspoon dried herb in hot water. Use 10 to 20 drops of the extract in warm water. Add 1 teaspoon of honey for a soothing drink.

Goldenseal* powder mixed in warm water relieves congestion and is soothing to inflamed mucous membranes. Use 1 teaspoon of goldenseal powder in 1 pint boiling water. Let cool. Take 1 to 2 teaspoons up to 6 times daily as needed. Or mix 5 to 10 drops extract in liquid, and take up to 3 times daily.

Lungwort* tea is good for upper respiratory problems and hoarseness. Lungwort is available in dried herb form. For tea, use 1 teaspoon dried herb in hot water. Drink 1 cup daily.

Mullein* tea is wonderful for dry, nagging coughs. Use 1 tablespoon of the dried herb in 1 cup hot water.

Drink up to 2 cups of this tea daily to relieve symptoms.

THE BEST HERBS FOR SORE THROATS

Fenugreek* gargle is excellent for sore, irritated throats. Use 20 drops of extract in 1 cup water. Gargle 3 times daily.

Slippery elm bark* lozenges help relieve throat pain.

Marshmallow* root tea is very soothing for scratchy, itchy throats. Use 1 teaspoon of the dried herb in 1 cup hot water. Drink up to 3 cups daily.

Raspberry* tea relieves pain due to sore throat. Raspberry tea is available in commercial preparations and dried herb. Use 1 teaspoon dried herb in 1 cup hot water. Drink 1 cup daily.

"JEWISH PENICILLIN"? IT CAN'T HURT

In the twelfth century, the great physician and philosopher Maimonides prescribed herbal baths and chicken soup as remedies for the common cold. Mothers have been following his advice ever since—at least the chicken soup part. More than eight hundred years later, the New England Journal of Medicine confirmed that Maimonides was right. Researchers found that chicken soup was a mild antibiotic and decongestant. To date, chicken soup is the only remedy that has been proven effective against the common cold. Chinese healers also use chicken soup to treat colds, but they add a little ginseng to their brew.

HERBS TO BRING DOWN A FEVER

White willow bark* helps break a fever. Take 2 capsules every 3 hours as needed.

Feverfew* is an old-time remedy to bring down a fever. Take 1 to 3 capsules until temperature is normal.

Barberry promotes sweating and helps to cool the body. Mix 3 to 7 drops of extract in ½ cup water. Drink up to 3 times daily.

HERBS FOR ALLERGIES

Ephedra* can help break up congestion due to hayfever. Take 1 to 3 capsules daily to relieve symptoms. This herb is also a long-acting stimulant. Do not use if you have high blood pressure.

Nettle* can relieve allergic symptoms such as teary eyes and runny nose. Take 1 to 2 tablets, up to 4 times daily as needed. Avoid this herb if you have high blood pressure.

An eyewash made from eyebright* is good for "allergic," itchy eyes. Mix 1 tablespoon herb in 1 cup hot water. Let cool. Use on eyes as needed.

HERBS THAT RELIEVE GAS AND INDIGESTION

Basil* is good for gassy stomach. Mix 1 teaspoon of dried herb in ½ cup warm water. Strain. Drink 1 to 2 cups daily.

Caraway* is a time-tested remedy for indigestion. Mix

3 to 4 drops of extract in 1 cup liquid. Drink 3 to 4 times daily as needed.

Catnip's* antispasmodic action is good for stomach cramps and helps you to relax. Mix ½ to 1 teaspoon extract in 1 cup liquid. Drink 1 to 2 cups daily.

Chamomile* tea is good for indigestion and has a calming effect on the body. Drink 1 cup nightly.

Dill* is excellent for gas and indigestion. Steep 2 teaspoons of dill seeds in 1 cup warm water for 10 to 15 minutes. Strain. Drink ½ cup up to 3 times daily.

Fennel* can relieve gas and cramps. Mix 10 to 20 drops of extract in 1 cup warm water. Sweeten with honey. Drink 2 to 3 cups as needed.

Papaya* tablets can help relieve indigestion. Take 1 tablet up to 3 times daily.

HERBAL REMEDIES FOR NAUSEA AND VOMITING

A cup of gingerroot* tea helps relieve nausea.

Peppermint* tea will quell stomach cramps and nausea.

Consuming 2 to 5 drops of clove* oil in ½ cup water will stop vomiting.

Cinnamon is excellent for upset stomach, gas, and diarrhea. Put a few drops of cinnamon oil in warm water. Drink as needed.

HERBS FOR CONSTIPATION

Cascara* is an excellent laxative for occasional problems. Cascara is available in capsule form. Do not exceed recommended dose.

Adding psyllium* to your diet will help keep you regular. Put 1 teaspoon in 1 cup water or juice, and drink 2 to 3 cups daily. Drink at least 8 glasses of water throughout the day.

HERBS TO STOP DIARRHEA AND CRAMPING

A grated, raw apple* (with the skin) is good for diarrhea.

Catnip* tea helps relieve diarrhea. Mix 1 tablespoon dried herb in 8 ounces hot water.

Arrowroot is good for an upset stomach. Mix 2 teaspoons in 2 cups warm water. Flavor with honey or cinnamon. Drink 2 cups daily.

Eating 3 grated, raw carrots* works well for diarrhea.

HERBS FOR WATER RETENTION AND BLOATING (DIURETICS)

Alfalfa* (tea or tablets) is a mild diuretic that is safe for just about everyone.

Juniper* berry is an excellent diuretic. Mix 10 to 20 drops of extract in 1 cup liquid. Take 2 to 3 times as needed.

HERBS FOR TOOTHACHE

Put 2 to 5 drops of clove* oil on affected area and call the dentist!

HERBAL MOUTHWASH

Barberry* strengthens weak gums. Mix 3 to 7 drops of extract in ½ cup water. Rinse 3 times daily.

A mouthwash made out of goldenseal* powder and water is excellent for sore gums and helps prevent gum disease.

Since biblical times, myrrh* has been used for irritated and infected gums and canker sores. Mix 2 to 5 drops in ½ cup water. Use as needed.

HERBAL MOISTURIZERS

Aloe gel* is one of the best! Use as needed.

Almond oil* is good for rough skin. Use as needed.

HERBS FOR SUNBURN

Gently rub any of these herbs on the burned area:

Cool chamomile* tea

Aloe gel*

Witch hazel*

HERBS FOR MINOR BURNS

Aloe gel* relieves pain and promotes healing of burns.

Honey (the kind you put in tea) is terrific for minor burns.

The juice from crushed gingeroot* relieves that hot, stinging sensation.

HERBS FOR SKIN IRRITATIONS

Arnica* lotion promotes healing of wounds. Use daily, only on unbroken skin!

Calendula* salve and ointment is soothing to skin wounds and bruises. Follow the directions on the package.

Comfrey* salve or ointment promotes healing of scrapes, cuts, and other skin wounds. Follow the directions on the package.

Elder* ointment is excellent for rashes. Follow the directions on the package.

Witch hazel is very soothing to skin inflammations. Use as needed.

Aloe gel* promotes healing of skin wounds. Use as needed.

HERBAL CURES FOR LICE AND ITCHING

Angelica* extract applied directly on irritated area kills lice and relieves itching. Use daily.

HERBS FOR RHEUMATISM, ARTHRITIS, AND MUSCLE ACHES

Eucalyptus* liniments are very soothing to sore, inflamed joints. Apply to affected area.

Used externally, angelica* extract is good for pain and swelling caused by rheumatism.

Turmeric,* a main ingredient of curry, is a well-known antiinflammatory that has been used for arthritis. Take 1 (300-mg) capsule up to 3 times daily.

Taken internally, chaparral* is reputed to be good for arthritis. Try 1 capsule for 3 times daily.

Fennel* oil rubbed on affected areas is an old-time remedy for rheumatism and arthritis.

An antiinflammatory, white willow bark* is used to relieve muscle aches and sprains, as well as arthritis. Take 2 capsules every 3 hours as needed.

HERBAL HEADACHE REMEDIES

Feverfew* helps prevent migraines. Take 1 capsule up to 3 times daily. It could take several months for you to see any improvement.

White willow bark* is an excellent aspirin substitute. Available in tablet form, take 2 capsules every 3 hours as needed.

A cup of peppermint* tea is soothing for a headache.

HERBS FOR DIZZINESS AND MOTION SICKNESS

Ginkgo* is excellent for chronic dizziness and light-headedness. Take 3 (40-mg) capsules daily.

Ginger* tablets or capsules are terrific for motion sickness. Take 1 capsule up to 3 times daily.

HERBS FOR EARACHES

A few drops of garlic* oil from a garlic capsule (a combination of garlic oil and other vegetable oils) can help an earache. (Undiluted garlic oil is too strong.)

Calendula* oil on a cotton swab can relieve an earache.

HERBAL BREATH FRESHENERS

Chew on a fresh parsley* sprig.

HERBAL DEODORANTS

Chlorella tablets help eliminate body odor. Take 1 to 3 daily.

HERBS FOR SKIN RASHES

Black walnut* extract is an old-time remedy for psoriasis. Try rubbing the extract directly on affected areas twice a day.

Goldenseal* is a folk cure for eczema. Rub extract on dry, red patches daily.

HERBS THAT PROMOTE SLEEP

A cup of chamomile* tea is very relaxing at night.

Siberian ginseng* is reputed to be a cure for insomnia. The herb is available in extract and capsules. Take

1 capsule up to 3 times daily or 5 to 10 drops of extract in 1 cup liquid daily.

HERBAL STRESS BUSTERS

Hops* is a relaxing herb. Mix ½ teaspoon in ½ cup water. Drink daily. Sprinkle hops on your pillow.

Passionflower* is especially good for times of acute anxiety. Mix 15 to 60 drops of extract in liquid. Drink daily. Do not use during pregnancy.

Valerian* is nature's own tranquilizer. Take 1 to 3 capsules daily, or 10 drops of extract in liquid.

Skullcap* is one of the oldest remedies for stress. Use 1 teaspoon of dried herb in 1 cup hot water for a home-brewed tea. Mix 3 to 12 drops of extract in liquid daily. Take 1 capsule up to 3 times daily.

HERBAL ENERGIZERS

Cayenne* has a mild stimulating effect. Try a cup of cayenne tea when you're feeling tired and run-down.

If used consistently, ginseng—Panax, American, or Siberian—can help eliminate fatigue. Ginseng is available in capsules, extract, or tea.

The Chinese herb schizandra is believed to increase energy and stamina.

Ephedra* (ma huang) is a long-acting stimulant. A cup of ephedra tea will perk you up.

HERBS FOR ATHLETE'S FOOT

Tea tree ointment or oil, which is sold in most health food stores, is excellent for this fungal infection. Follow the directions on the package.

Apple cider vinegar is an old folk remedy for athlete's foot. Rub on affected areas several times a day. (It might sting a little at first, but persevere; it is effective.)

CHAPTER 6

A Woman's Body

Modern medicine has been a predominantly male profession. In fact, it was only within the past decade that medical schools began admitting women in equal numbers with men. Ironically, however, the first healers were probably women, and the drugs they used were the seeds, leaves, berries, and bark they collected for food. It's not surprising that women would take such an active interest in healing. Their unique biology and hormonal cycles—the fact that they menstruate and bear children—made it all the more important for them to have a basic understanding of herbal medicine. Unfortunately, much of this knowledge has been lost and the rich tradition of the "wise woman healer" is fast becoming a thing of the past. Women are constantly asking me about natural alternatives to the drugs and procedures that are typically used for female complaints. Here are some of the questions that women commonly ask me about herbs. *Note*: Herbs that are listed in the "Hot Hundred" are designated by an asterisk (*). Please refer to "Hot Hundred" entries for more information.

MENOPAUSE

Since I've recently become menopausal, I have suffered from frequent hot flashes that make me very uncomfortable. My doctor suggested that I try estrogen replacement therapy, but I read that estrogen can increase your risk of developing cancer. Are there any herbs that I can try instead?

The sudden drop in estrogen levels is responsible for many of the annoying symptoms that women experience during menopause, including hot flashes, mood swings, and headaches. Most of these symptoms disappear on their own within a year or two, but for some women, it can be a year or two of pure torture. Fortunately, there are several herbs that can help. Many women find that ginseng* can greatly relieve the hot flashes and other unpleasant side effects associated with the change of life. Try 1 capsule up to 3 times daily or 1 cup of ginseng tea every day. In rare cases, ginseng may stimulate vaginal bleeding, which in this case is harmless, but it can be quite frightening. Any kind of vaginal bleeding after menstruation may be a warning sign of cancer and should be reported immediately to your physician. However, make sure that your physician knows that you've been using ginseng.

Chinese women use dong quai*—often called the "female ginseng"—to help smooth the transition to menopause. Dong quai is highly regarded as a tonic for the female sex organs and is reported to be good for vaginal dryness, another problem associated with menopause. Try 1 capsule up to 3 times daily. Vitex (*Agnus castus*) is another herb that is becoming popular in Europe for problems associated with the menstrual cycle, including menopause. Vitex capsules are available at many health food stores. You may want to try each of these herbs for two weeks to see which works best for you. In addition, a few of the major herb companies have special formulas designed specifically for menopausal women. These preparations may include such as pennyroyal,* black cohosh,* dong quai,* valerian,* and licorice. These formulas are designed to help women cope with the physical and emotional stresses of menopause and many women I've spoken with say they are excellent.

CAUTION

Women with high blood pressure should not take any herbal preparation containing licorice.*

PREMENSTRUAL SYNDROME

About ten days before my period is due, I suffer from terrible PMS. I get very cranky, my breasts become very sore, and I feel exhausted. Is there anything that can help?

You're not alone. As many as 50 percent of all women may experience some form of premenstrual syndrome including excessive water retention, headaches, mood swings, and breast tenderness. PMS disappears once menstruation begins. For some women, the symptoms are very minor and can be ignored. For other women, however, this is not the case, and like you, they spend a week or more each month in great discomfort. For these women, I recommend evening primrose oil.* Several carefully conducted studies performed in London and Canada of women with severe PMS show that the majority of women studied experienced a marked reduction in symptoms after being treated with evening primrose oil. For best results, take 3 (250-mg) capsules daily starting three days prior to the usual onset of PMS symptoms until menstruation.

If evening primrose oil doesn't work for you, try either dong quai* or vitex capsules, which are also popular treatments. In addition, during the time of the month that you are most vulnerable to retaining water, avoid salty food. Try eating herbs with natural diuretic properties such as alfalfa,* asparagus,* celery,* dandelion,* and carrot.* Avoid excess caffeine, which could make you jittery. End the day with a relaxing cup of chamomile* tea. You should notice a difference in how you feel almost immediately.

REGULATING MENSTRUATION AFTER BIRTH CONTROL PILLS

I've been taking birth control pills for five years and now want to stop. I understand that it could take several months for my menstrual cycle to return to normal and I'm worried about getting pregnant and not knowing it. Is there any herb that I should be taking during this transition period to promote normal menstruation?

Women herbalists recommend dong quai* to help restore normal hormonal patterns in women who have taken birth control pills. (This herb should not be used during pregnancy or if you have excessive menstrual flow.)

MENSTRUAL CRAMPS

I suffer from bad menstrual cramps and am allergic to ibuprofen, the drug usually prescribed by doctors for this problem. Are there any herbal alternatives?

Fortunately, you have several excellent herbal options. False unicorn, known as the uterine tonic, is available in dried form and can be made into a soothing tea. Valerian,* nature's own tranquilizer, can also help relieve uterine cramping. It is available in tea, extract, and capsules. Dong quai,* pennyroyal,* and vitex are also used for menstrual cramps and are widely available in easy-to-use preparations. For cramping and headache, try white willow* capsules, a pain reliever that is similar to aspirin but less irritating to the stomach. In addition, many herb manufacturers have special formulas in capsule form designed to relieve menstrual cramps. Chamomile* tea is an age-old remedy for cramping. Try one or more of these herbs to see which works the best for you.

CHRONIC YEAST INFECTION

I suffer from a recurrent vaginal yeast infection that is quite annoying. When I have an active case, my doctor prescribes a cream that works right away to relieve the itchiness and discomfort, but a month or two later the infection is back. Do you have any suggestions?

Yeast is actually a minute fungus, and therefore, there are some herbs with antifungal properties that I think could be of help. Studies show that pau d'arco,* a South American herb, has been used successfully against parasites and is lethal to fungus. Pau d'arco is available in capsule form. Odorless garlic* capsules may also help prevent a recurrence. For centuries, women have used a douche made out of goldenseal* to cure all kinds of vaginal infections, including yeast. It's certainly worth a try. (Goldenseal should not be used during pregnancy.) In the *Vitamin Bible*, I recommend taking acidophilus tablets or capsules (milk free) for yeast infections and eating yogurt with active cultures.

"RESTLESS LEG SYNDROME"

My legs are driving me crazy! When I'm sitting still, they feel achy and stiff. As a result, I am constantly squirming and moving around. My doctor called it "restless leg syndrome" and told me that it is quite common among women. He had no other advice to give. Is there anything I can do about it?

Restless leg syndrome, also known as heavy leg syndrome, is caused by poor circulation. Several European studies show that many women with this problem find relief from butcher's broom,* an herb that is widely available in capsule and extract form. Although this herb is not generally used by doctors in the United States, it is widely prescribed in Europe.

VARICOSE VEINS AND HEMORRHOIDS

I'm a dental hygienist, and I spend most of the day on my feet. Although I wear support hose, I am still bothered by varicose veins. The veins on my legs are swollen and sore, especially at night. Are there any herbs that I should be using?

Varicose veins are veins that have become swollen and enlarged. They occur more often in women than men, and frequently are a result of pregnancy. Hemorrhoids are swollen or varicose anal veins. Varicose veins are a sign of poor circulation. In your case, standing on your feet all day is allowing the blood to pool in your legs, resulting in the varicosity. There are several time-honored remedies that are quite popular in Europe. Butcher's broom,* which is used to improve overall circulation, has been shown to greatly relieve both varicose veins and hemorrhoids. For hemorrhoids, it is available in suppository form. Horse chestnut* is another herb that is very soothing to inflamed veins. Available in powder form in the United States, it can be diluted with warm water and gently rubbed on sore veins and hemorrhoids. (Mix ½ teaspoon powder to 16 ounces water.) Applied externally, witch hazel will help reduce some of the discomfort caused by varicose veins and hemorrhoids.

EPISIOTOMY

I'm pregnant with my second child. During my first pregnancy, the worst part of labor and delivery was the episiotomy. The procedure was painful enough, but what really bothered me was the fact that it took forever to heal. If I have to have an episiotomy again, is there anything I can do to hasten the healing process?

An episiotomy is a surgical incision of the vulva to prevent tearing during the second stage of labor. I have heard from many women that the pain from the episiotomy can linger for several weeks and even months. There is an herb that may help. According to a 1966 study in a French obstetrical journal, extract of gotu kola*—sometimes called centella—helped to promote healing after episiotomy. The study noted that the women who used centella extract immediately after the procedure reported less pain and faster healing than those who had been given standard medication. The doctors in the study said that for best results centella should be used as early in the procedure as possible. Gotu kola or centella extract is easily available in most health food stores or herb shops. Obviously, you'll need your doctor's cooperation, so talk to him or her about using centella ahead of time.

IRREGULAR PERIODS, MISSED PERIODS

My menstrual periods are very irregular and sometimes disappear for months at a time. Are there any herbs that can help regulate my period?

There are several herbs that are used to regulate the menstrual cycle. Blessed thistle* is one of the oldest folk remedies for amenorrhea, the absence of menstruation after the onset of the menstrual cycle. Blessed thistle is available in capsule and extract forms. Dong quai,* which is used for many gynecological problems, is also reputed to normalize the menstrual cycle. Pennyroyal* is another herb that has historically been used to promote menstruation. (Neither don quai nor pennyroyal should be used during pregnancy. Pennyroyal is sometimes used by herbal healers during labor and delivery.)

MORNING SICKNESS

Since I became pregnant, I wake up every morning feeling nauseous. Sometimes I feel sick to my stomach again late in the afternoon. I'm afraid to take any antinausea medication because I don't want to hurt the baby. Any suggestions?

You have a classic case of morning sickness, a misnomer because it can strike anytime during the day, especially when you're feeling fatigued. To get rid of that nauseous feeling, drink a cup of gingeroot* tea or take 1 ginger tablet or capsule first thing in the morning. During the day, alternate between drinking ginger ale and peppermint* tea. None of these simple remedies will hurt your baby, and you'll feel a whole lot better.

LABOR AND DELIVERY

I'm working with a midwife and would like to avoid taking painkillers during labor and delivery. What did women do before meperidine and epidurals?

In the old days, before high-tech delivery rooms, women prepared for labor on their own. Starting at about the eighth month, they would sip several cups of raspberry* tea throughout the day to tone their uterus for labor. During labor, they used herbs such as pennyroyal,* blue cohosh,* and raspberry* leaves to promote uterine contractions. Although these herbs may not have reduced the pain, they may have helped to expedite labor, which is half the battle. Talk to your midwife about having an "herbal delivery."

NURSING

I want to nurse my baby but am having trouble producing enough milk. What herbs are good for nursing mothers?

For centuries, dill* and anise* have been used to promote milk production in nursing mothers. In fact, a recent study shows that just the smell of anise promotes milk production in cows! For best results, steep 2 teaspoons of dill seed in 1 warm cup water for 10 to 15 minutes. Take ½ cup 2 to 3 times a day. To use anise seed, mix 1 teaspoon in 1 cup warm water. Drink up to 3 times daily.

FEMALE TONICS

Are there herbs that are beneficial to the female reproductive system? Are there such things as aphrodisiacs?

Dong quai,* which is used for a number of gynecological problems, is also used as an overall female tonic. Damiana* is considered a sexual tonic for both men and women and is reputed to be an aphrodisiac, although there is no scientific evidence to back up this claim. In fact, although people have talked about aphrodisiacs for centuries, there is no hard scientific evidence to prove that they really exist. In folk medicine, however, asparagus* and artichokes* are highly regarded as aphrodisiacs for both sexes.

ANEMIA

Are there any herbs that can help prevent iron-deficiency anemia?

I would recommend two herbs—nettle* and chives.* They are both rich in vitamin C and iron, a perfect combination since vitamin C facilitates the body's absorption of iron. Iron is essential for the formation of red blood cells. Chives should be eaten fresh, but fresh nettle can be dangerous. Therefore, stick to extract, capsules, or dried herb, which are perfectly safe in the recommended dose.

OVARIAN CANCER

I recently read about an herb called taxol that was being touted as a cure of ovarian cancer. Can you tell me more about it?

Taxol is an extract of the Pacific yew tree. Recent clinical trials have shown taxol to be effective in cases of ovarian cancer that did not respond to conventional treatment. Unfortunately, according to a leading pharmacy magazine, taxol is in short supply due to an ever-diminishing number of yew trees. In fact, environmental groups in the Northwest are fighting to prevent these trees from being cut down by loggers and developers.

OSTEOPOROSIS

Now that I'm nearing menopause, my doctor warned me that I was at greater risk of developing osteoporosis. What should I be doing to prevent this?

Osteoporosis is a condition in which bones become thin and brittle, leaving them prone to fractures and breaks. This potentially debilitating disease is more common among postmenopausal women, which has led researchers to believe that falling estrogen levels are somehow responsible for the weakening of the bones. Synthetic estrogens are often given to prevent further bone loss. Eating a diet high in calcium may help prevent osteoporosis. In addition to dairy products, broccoli, kale, almonds,* and collard greens are excellent sources of this vital mineral. I also recommend taking horsetail* (silica), an herb that helps the body absorb and utilize calcium. Take 1 capsule or tablet up to 3 times daily.

CHAPTER 7

A Man's Body

Here are some answers to questions that I am frequently asked by men about herbal remedies for common male complaints. *Note*: Herbs that are listed in the "Hot Hundred" are designated by an asterisk (*). Refer to the "Hot Hundred" for more information.

ENLARGED PROSTATE

I recently went to my doctor for a checkup because I have to urinate very frequently, especially at night. My doctor told me that I have an enlarged prostate, which he said was not very serious. In fact, he did not even offer any treatment. Are there any herbs that can help?

The prostate is a group of small glands that surround the urethra at the point where it leaves the bladder. Although we don't know exactly what the prostate does, it secretes a fluid that is believed to stimulate the movement of sperm after ejaculation. Nearly every man over forty-five has some form of prostate enlargement and, in most cases, it is a harmless condition. However, due to its location near the urethra, a sufficiently enlarged prostate can cause urinary problems. Any change in urinary patterns should be brought to the attention of your doctor. If urine is not passing properly, there is a greater risk of kidney infection or cystitis.

An enlarged prostate can also be a sign of other problems, including cancer. If the outflow of urine is blocked, treatment including surgery may be necessary. However, in most cases, an enlarged prostate is a benign albeit annoying condition. In fact, as in your case, you may be told to simply live with it. There are some herbs that are reputed to be good for prostate problems. In Germany, saw palmetto* is a highly regarded treatment for mild prostate conditions, although it is not recognized as a legitimate treatment in the United States. Saw palmetto is available here in extract form. Take 30 to 60 drops in 1 cup liquid daily until the condition improves. Uva ursi* (bearberry) is another time-honored remedy for urinary tract problems. Take 1 to 3 capsules daily to relieve symptoms. In addition, avoid caffeinated drinks and alcohol, and try not to drink too much liquid before going to bed.

PERSISTENT FUNGAL INFECTION

Since I've joined a gym, I have developed a chronic fungus infection on my feet, which is extremely uncomfortable. My doctor gave me some antifungal pills, but they made me very nauseous. Is there anything else I can do?

A fungus is a microscopic plantlike organism that likes to take up residence on the human body. It's not surprising that you developed this problem after joining the gym—you probably picked it up in the shower or in the communal dressing areas. There are a few herbs that can help strengthen your resistance against fungal infections. Pau d'arco* is one of them. Studies show that this South American herb has antifungal, antiparasitic properties. Take 3 capsules daily. Garlic* is another herb that may help your body ward off these troublesome pests. Take 1 to 3 odorless garlic capsules daily. To relieve the dry, itchy feeling, use an ointment containing tea tree oil, a natural fungicide. Keep your feet as dry as possible and change your socks often. Some herbalists recommend sprinkling a mixture of goldenseal* powder and talcum powder on your feet to absorb moisture and kill the fungus. Fungal infections are very persistent, and it may take several weeks (or even months) before you get relief.

PREMATURE BALDNESS

The men in my family tend to go bald at an early age. I'm thirty-five, still have a full head of hair, and want to keep it that way! Are there any herbs that can help prevent hair loss?

Before I get your hopes up, it's important to note that patterns of hair loss are largely determined by genetics. Therefore, there are few legitimate remedies for baldness. In some cases, a sluggish thyroid or other medical problem may trigger hair loss, and once treated, the condition will very often reverse itself. There are some herbs that are reputed to prevent signs of premature aging, such as baldness, but these claims have not been scientifically investigated. However, they're certainly worth a try. The Chinese swear that fo-ti,* a popular tonic herb in the Orient, prevents gray hair and other signs of aging. Take 1 capsule up to 3 times daily. Herbalists also recommend massaging the scalp with an extract of rosemary prior to the onset of hair loss. After the treatment, shampoo as usual.

IMPOTENCE

I've heard a lot about herbal aphrodisiacs, and I wonder, is there an herb that can help impotence?

For centuries, the bark of the yohimbe tree has been used as a treatment for impotency in Africa. In fact, the drug yohimbine, an extract of this herb, is recognized as a legitimate treatment for impotency in the United States. However, yohimbine is potentially toxic to the liver and can cause a sudden decline in blood pressure. Therefore, it should only be used under the supervision of a qualified physician, if at all. Anyone who is suffering from chronic impotency should consult a doctor. The problem could be physical in origin, such as hormonal imbalance, or it could be a result of excessive stress or other psychological factors. In either case, treatment may be necessary. However, if the problem is only occasional, there are some herbs that may help. Damiana* is reputed to be a tonic for sexual organs and is safe to take on a daily basis. Take up to 3 capsules daily. The Chinese herb schizandra is also supposed to enhance sexual performance in men and is also safe for long-term use. Take up to 3 capsules daily.

INCREASE STAMINA

I have begun working out on a regular basis and want to know if there is anything I can take to improve my performance. I know someone who is taking steroids and it really seems to help, but I hear that they can be dangerous. Are there any herbal alternatives?

First, I want to caution you to steer clear of steroids. Synthetic steroids are potent drugs that have many serious side effects, including death. In teenage boys, these drugs can interfere with normal sexual development. Steroids also depress the immune system, which will leave you more vulnerable to infection. In addition, they can cause fluid retention, high blood pressure, and other serious medical problems. Although they may increase muscle mass, they do not increase strength. Many weight lifters who rely on steroids for their brawny appearance may deceive themselves into thinking that they are stronger than they are. As a result, they may routinely overexert themselves, which can result in serious injury. Steroids are simply not worth the risk.

Fortunately, there are some herbs that can help improve physical performance. Studies show that so-called adaptogen herbs popular in China, such as ginseng* and schizandra, can help the body better withstand the stress of physical exertion. In order to reap the full benefits from these herbs, they should be used daily. (They are both available in capsule form. Follow the directions on the package.) Some bodybuilders swear that sarsaparilla* helps increase muscle mass, although there is no scientific evidence to support this claim. It's certainly worth a try, and is a lot safer than steroids. Sarsaparilla is available in capsules: Take up to 3 daily.

MUSCLE STRAINS

I'm a weekend athlete who frequently wakes up on a Monday morning with sore, aching muscles. Any suggestions?

Arnica* ointment is excellent for overworked muscles. Follow the directions on the package. However, don't use it on broken skin—it can be very irritating. Eucalyptus* ointment can also help by promoting blood flow to the sore areas, producing a feeling of warmth. Use several times daily as needed. In addition, white willow bark,* an herbal aspirin substitute, can reduce pain and inflammation. Take 2 tablets every 3 to 4 hours as needed.

AFTER-SHAVE RASH

I have sensitive skin. Frequently, after I shave, my face erupts in a tiny, red rash that is very annoying. Are there any herbal products that could help?

Witch hazel is very soothing for minor skin irritations. Splash it on immediately after shaving. Calendula* ointment is also excellent for sore spots. Apply after shaving. In addition, use an aloe* cream daily to help restore moisture and promote healing.

CHAPTER 8

Herbal Preventive Medicine

For more than five thousand years, herbal practitioners have understood the simple fact that diet and lifestyle can have a profound effect on health. Until very recently, doctors who espoused this philosophy were considered radical or were dismissed as practitioners of holistic medicine. It has only been within the past decade that the medical profession grudgingly accepted the link between a high-fat diet and a whole host of ailments, including cancer and heart disease. And it has only been within the past few years that leading cancer researchers have finally begun to investigate the possibility of using potent antitumor chemicals found in fruits and vegetables to prevent cancer. While the medical profession has been dragging its feet, natural healers have been using herbs to promote wellness and prevent disease. Here is a list of some herbs that can help maintain health and vigor. *Note*: Herbs that are described in the "Hot Hundred" are designated with an asterisk (*). For information on how to use these herbs, please check the "Hot Hundred" listing.

FOODS THAT FIGHT CANCER

The National Cancer Institute is investigating the possibility of using highly concentrated forms of anticarcinogenic plant chemicals in foods designed specifically to help prevent cancer. Researchers are considering using several plant compounds in these "designer foods," including high levels of indoles from the cabbage family, which prevent the growth of certain estrogen-sensitive tumors, and antitumor compounds found in garlic and rosemary. Within a few years, supermarket shelves may be filled with fortified foods engineered to prevent specific forms of cancer. For example, there could be a cereal targeted for women who are at risk of developing breast cancer, and another for people who are concerned about colon cancer.

HERBS FOR A HEALTHY HEART

Evening primrose oil* can reduce cholesterol. In one 1983 study performed by researchers at the Efamol Research Institute in Canada, patients with high cholesterol who took evening primrose oil for three months averaged more than a 30 percent drop in cholesterol levels. This herb has also been shown to lower blood pressure.

For centuries, Chinese doctors have used ginseng* as a heart tonic. Numerous studies have documented what the Chinese knew all along: ginseng lowers cholesterol, lowers blood sugar, and normalizes blood pressure.

In animal studies, cayenne* has reduced triglycerides and LDLs, the so-called bad cholesterol carrier in the blood. Elevated triglycerides (over 190 mg) are a major risk factor for heart disease in women.

Artichoke* reduces cholesterol. The anticholesterol drug cynara is a derivative of this plant.

Garlic* is a terrific "cholesterol buster." It raises HDL (the good cholesterol), lowers LDL (the bad cholesterol), and reduces triglycerides. Elevated triglycerides in women (over 190 mg/dl) is considered a major risk factor for developing coronary artery disease.

Ever wonder why heart disease is relatively rare in Mediterranean countries? It could be that the people in these countries consume a lot more olive oil* than we do in the United States. Recent studies show that olive oil, a highly monounsaturated fat, lowers overall blood cholesterol without reducing the beneficial HDLs. Sprinkle a tablespoon or two of olive oil in your salad daily instead of other oils.

Oat* bran is rich in beta glucan, a water-soluble form of fiber. Two ounces of oats daily in a low-fat diet can reduce blood cholesterol levels by 5 to 10 percent.

Studies show that the husks of the psyllium* plant (the active ingredient in the over-the-counter laxative, Metamucil) can lower cholesterol in men with moderately high cholesterol levels. (Women were not included in the tests, but that doesn't mean that it won't work for them, too!) Some people who use this herb have allergic reactions, so watch for any allergic symptoms, including respiratory problems or a rash.

HERBS THAT MAY HELP PREVENT CANCER

Triterpenoids, chemicals found in licorice* root, appear to prevent some precancerous cells from developing abnormally. The cancer-fighting properties of triterpenoids are currently being investigated by the National Cancer Institute. Triterpenoids deactivate certain kinds of potentially lethal estrogens in the body that are responsible for some forms of estrogen-sensitive breast tumors and other cancerous growths.

Recent studies performed by researchers at the Institute for Hormone Research in New York suggest that the vegetables in the cabbage family, such as broccoli, cauliflower, and bok choy, contain potent anticancer chemicals. These vegetables are rich in indoles, compounds that convert certain potentially carcinogenic estrogens into a benign form that will not trigger the growth of estrogen-sensitive tumors. The Institute for Hormone Research is investigating the cancer-fighting potential of certain foods.

People who eat diets high in alliums (garlic* and onions*) have significantly lower rates of cancer than those who don't.

Eating one raw carrot* a day can reduce your risk of getting certain forms of cancer. Cancer researchers have found that eating 12,500 IU of beta carotene daily (there are 13,500 IU in one raw carrot) can prevent certain forms of cancer, such as cancer of the esophagus, stomach, intestines, and prostate.

Shiitake mushroom* is used as a cancer-fighting treatment in Japan and China.

HERBS THAT PROMOTE GOOD CIRCULATION

The incidence of blood clots in countries that routinely use curry in their cuisines is much lower than in the United States. Herbs such as turmeric,* garlic,* cayenne*—usual ingredients in curry powder—are believed to help prevent platelets from sticking together and forming dangerous blood clots that could result in heart attack and stroke.

Studies show that extract of ginkgo* helps improve the blood supply throughout the body, especially to the brain. A 1980 French study shows that ginkgo prevents cells from sticking together to form dangerous blood clots, which could impair the flow of blood and cause stroke and heart attack.

HERBS THAT COUNTERACT THE EFFECTS OF AGING

Chaparral* prevents the formation of free radicals, compounds that disrupt normal cell function and are believed to cause certain forms of cancer and premature aging.

The Chinese consider the herb fo-ti* to be a rejuvenating tonic. Oriental herbalists claim that it prevents gray hair and signs of premature aging. Recent Chinese studies suggest that the herb can inhibit the growth of certain types of cancerous tumors and also helps prevent blood clots.

Ginkgo* extract, which promotes the flow of blood to

the brain, can help increase mental alertness in elderly people. In a recent German study, one group of elderly patients was given extract of ginkgo and another group was given a placebo. Those given ginkgo showed an improvement in mental reaction time and were more alert than those who took the placebo. Those who had the slowest mental reaction time prior to taking ginkgo showed the greatest improvement after being given the ginkgo extract.

HERBAL IMMUNE BOOSTERS

Studies show that the Chinese herb astragalus* enhances the body's ability to fight against cancer cells and viruses. It is being investigated as a possible treatment for AIDS.

Echinacea,* an herb introduced to the settlers by Native Americans, has been shown to be a potent immune booster, strengthening the body's ability to ward off invading infections.

To strengthen your immune system, stick to oriental cuisines. Garlic,* shiitake,* and reishi mushrooms (included in the section on up-and-coming herbs on page 170) help prevent the growth of tumors and increase the body's ability to fight unwanted invaders.

HERBS FOR THE LIVER

Milk thistle* helps regenerate liver cells and helps cleanse the liver of dangerous toxins. In several European studies performed in the 1970s on rats, animals who had their livers partially removed experienced a regeneration of liver cells after receiving milk thistle extract.

In 1940, a Japanese researcher discovered that artichoke* stimulates the production of bile and may protect against jaundice and other disorders related to the liver. Dandelion,* another traditional remedy for liver disorders, is rich in lecithin, a substance that researchers recently discovered may protect against cirrhosis of the liver.

Turmeric* increases the production of bile and may help reduce inflammation of the liver. Since 1936, numerous European and Indian studies have confirmed turmeric's protective effect on the liver.

HERBS FOR VISION

Bilberry* protects eyesight by accelerating the production of retinal purple, a substance that is critical for good vision.

BOTANICAL SOURCES OF VITAMINS

Vitamin A
Alfalfa, annatto, dandelion, okra, paprika, parsley, kelp, watercress.

B-Complex
Apples, bananas, beans, beets, cabbage, carrots, cauliflower, corn, grapefruit, kelp, mushrooms, onions, oranges, peas, peanuts, potatoes, raisins, spinach, strawberries, tomatoes, turnips, wheat, whole seeds, yeast.

Vitamin C
All green and citrus fruits, rose hips, black currants, red currants, strawberries, potatoes, spinach, cabbage, watercress, turnips.

Vitamin D
Annatto, watercress, wheat germ, all oil-containing seeds.

Vitamin E
All seeds, alfalfa, oats, flax, sesame, wheat germ, soybeans, green leafy vegetables, dulse, kelp, watercress.

Vitamin K
Alfalfa, chestnut leaves.

BOTANICAL SOURCES OF OTHER NUTRIENTS

Unsaturated Fatty Acids
Unsaturated fatty acids are produced by plants and are important for normal cell function. There are two kinds of unsaturated fatty acids: polyunsaturates and monounsaturates. Polyunsaturates contain linoleic acid, a critical ingredient in the formation of cells and the functioning of the nervous system. Monounsaturates contain oleic acid, and have been shown to lower blood cholesterol levels when used in place of saturated fats from animal or dairy sources. Foods that are rich in unsaturated fatty acids include: barley, coconut, peanuts, rapeseed, linseed, corn, oats, olives, rice, rye, soybeans, sunflower seeds, wheat.

Bioflavonoids
Bioflavonoids (also called vitamin P) refer to a group of biologically active substances found in plants that offer many benefits. Flavonoids often work in conjunction with vitamin C. Two flavonoids, quercetin and catechin, are potent antioxidants that prevent the formation of free radicals, substances that are believed to cause premature aging and certain types of cancer. Quercetin is well known for its antitumor properties. In general, flavonoids are beneficial to the cardiovascular system and help strengthen the immune system. Foods that are rich in flavonoids include: apples, beets, blackberries, black currants, cabbage, carrots, cauliflower, cherries, dandelions, lemons, lentils, lettuce, oranges, paprika, parsley, peas, plums, potatoes, rhubarb, rose hips, spinach, turnips, tomatoes, walnuts, watercress.

CHAPTER 9

Looking Good

Whether you're a man or a woman, looking good goes hand in hand with feeling good. Before you read this chapter, however, I must caution that there is nothing on earth that can mask the ravages of an unhealthy lifestyle. The results of a lifetime of smoking, too much drinking, too little exercise, and a poor diet cannot be hidden under makeup or washed away by a scrub. The proper nutrition, the right vitamins, regular exercise, and sufficient sleep are the most important ingredients for staying attractive. Once you're living right, herbal preparations can help keep you looking your best.

Popular shops such as The Body Shop, Crabtree and Evelyn, and L'Herbier de Province, a newcomer to the United States, are filled with wonderful herbal grooming products. In fact, just about any herbal skin or hair product can be found in a packaged form. However, making your own can be fun. Best of all, you can tailor your grooming aids to suit your specific needs.

HERBS FOR HAIR

Regimen for Dry Hair

Everybody wants strong, shiny, lustrous hair, but dry hair is often brittle and dull. A warm oil conditioner can help replenish some of the natural oils that are depleted by too much sun, hair dryers, and hair spray. This preparation is also an excellent dandruff treatment. Mix one cup of extra virgin olive oil (use a mildly scented, light oil) with ½ cup dried rosemary leaves. Warm on top of the stove in small pot. Remove from heat and let the mixture cool to a comfortable, warm temperature. Use a comb to separate your hair, and apply oil to dry scalp and hair with a cotton ball. Make sure to cover the entire scalp. Put a shower cap over your hair, and then cover with a turban made out of thin towel. Let the oil soak in for about 30 minutes. Wash out thoroughly with a mild, herbal shampoo. It will take several lathers to remove the oil. Do not use an additional conditioner—you don't need it. Repeat treatment monthly. Your hair will be shiny and more manageable.

Quick Rinse for Dry Hair

Brew 2 cups of marshmallow tea. Let cool. Rinse through after shampoo.

Regimen for Oily Hair

Overzealous oil glands can leave hair stringy and limp. Horsetail (silica) is the herb to use to control excess oil production and to bring life back to listless, uncooperative hair. There are several commercial hair products available in health food stores that contain horsetail or silica. Your best bet is to use one of them. Horsetail is also available in capsule form and is reputed to strengthen weak hair strands. Take 1 to 3 capsules daily.

Rinse to Bring Out Blond Highlights

Since the days of the Roman Empire, chamomile has been used to put golden highlights back into light-colored hair. For an excellent highlighting rinse (that's good enough to drink), put 2 tablespoons chamomile dried herb into 16 ounces of hot water. Simmer ½ hour. Add the juice of 1 small lemon. After you shampoo, lean over the sink, and pour herbal mixture through hair slowly, making sure that the entire head of hair is covered. Catch remaining fluid in a bowl. Let mixture stand on hair 1 minute and then pour remaining fluid over hair. (Be sure to avoid your eyes; the lemon will make them sting.) Rinse out thoroughly with warm water. Repeat weekly. You'll notice a real difference in your hair, especially in the sunlight.

Rinse for Dark Hair

If you want to bring out a rich, dark sheen, try this recipe. Make 2 cups of regular, dark tea. (You can use a commercial tea bag.) Add 2 tablespoons dried rosemary leaves. Let simmer for 30 minutes. After you shampoo, lean over the sink, and pour herbal mixture through hair slowly, catching the remaining fluid in a bowl. Let mixture stay on hair for about a minute, and pour remaining fluid over hair. Massage mixture into hair. Rinse thoroughly with warm water. Repeat weekly.

Rinse to Rid Hair of Shampoo Residue

After shampooing, a vinegar rinse is the best way to wash out any shampoo buildup that can make the hair look dull. Put ¼ cup dried rosemary and ½ cup dried peppermint in a bowl and set aside. Put 2 cups of clear apple cider vinegar in a pot. Warm vinegar mixture on stove until it almost reaches boiling point. Pour vinegar over herbs. Let cool. Pour into a plastic container and let stand for one week, shaking the mixture daily. Strain mixture through a double layer of cheesecloth and add a few drops of a nicely scented essential oil to mask the vinegar smell. After washing your hair, mix ½ cup of herbal vinegar to 3 to 4 cups water, and pour mixture over hair as final rinse. Use weekly to avoid excess shampoo residue.

Herbs to Prevent Premature Gray

Fo ti—a highly popular herb in China—is reputed to prevent signs of premature aging such as gray hair. I don't know for a fact whether this is true, but it seems to me that Chinese people usually go gray much later in life than Caucasians—and many retain full heads of dark hair well into old age. Try it and see!

Approximately 120 years ago, this concoction was believed to promote hair growth.

> 3 quarts rum
> 1 pint spirit of wine
> 1 pint water
> ½ ounce extract of catharides (Spanish flies)
> ½ ounce carbonate of ammonia
> 1 ounce salt of tartar

Mix ingredients in a bowl. Rub well on hair. Rinse with water.

EYE CARE

Tired, worn-out–looking eyes can make you look old before your time. Fatigue, pollution, and allergies are all possible causes of red, sore eyes. To give tired eyes a lift, place fresh cucumber slices over each eye. Lie down in a dark room for 30 minutes. Your eyes will look and feel less sore and puffy. Beware of using commercial eyedrops. Frequent use of these over-the-counter products can result in chronic eye irritation. If you need to use an eyewash, try eyebright. Mix 2 tablespoons of the herb in 16 ounces hot water. Let cool. Strain. Use a small cup to pour mixture into each eye, or apply to each eye with a clean cotton ball. (Do not use the same cotton ball for both eyes, as this may spread the infection.)

HERBS FOR STRONG NAILS

If your nails are constantly peeling and chipping, or if they have white spots, you need to include more calcium in your diet. Eat more broccoli, collard greens, and low-fat dairy products. In addition, take a horsetail (silica) supplement, which facilitates the absorption of calcium by the body.

If your nails are dry and splitting, and your cuticles are ragged, a hot oil treatment can be very beneficial. Warm ½ cup almond oil in a small pot. (Don't let it get too hot.) Pour into a bowl and soak the fingertips on each hand for about 15 minutes. Rub remaining oil into cuticles, hands, and on the soles of the feet for a smooth, satiny feeling.

HERBS FOR SKIN CARE

Regimen for Dry, Itchy Skin

People with dry skin should avoid exposure to harsh soaps and detergents, which will further deplete the body of its natural, protective oils. Stick to unscented, superfatted soaps made out of natural ingredients including cocoa butter, aloe, jojoba oil, and wheat germ oil. After showering or bathing, always use a moisturizer to avoid that dry, tight feeling. Aloe and jojoba products are good choices. During the cold months, moisturize twice daily. For dry, flaky patches of skin, use evening primrose oil. Rub on the affected areas 1 to 2 times daily. Evening primrose oil is rich in linoleic acid, an essential fatty acid. People on low-fat diets may find that their skin is drier than usual and that they need additional lubrication. Rubbing evening primrose oil on their skin can help restore some of the lost oil.

Chapped Hands

Many people suffer from chapped hands, especially in the winter. To avoid irritation, wear cotton-lined rubber gloves when you wash dishes or do other household chores. In addition, for an excellent, old-fashioned hand cream—the kind that kept your grandmother's hands silky soft—mix ½ cup rosewater with ½ cup glycerin. Store in a plastic or glass jar. Rub on hands as needed.

At-Home Herbal Steam Facial

For just a few dollars' worth of herbs, you can give yourself the kind of steam facial typical of the swanky spas. It's easy to do, very relaxing, and a great way to deep clean clogged pores. Boil 1 quart of water. Mix in 2 tablespoons of yarrow, 2 tablespoons of lavender, 1 tablespoon of peppermint, and 1 tablespoon of fennel seeds. (Comfrey root, chamomile, and orange blossoms can be substituted for any of the above ingredients.) Put pot in a low sink or on a table. Stand about 1 foot away. Make a tentlike cover out of towel and hold it over your head as you lean over the hot pot. Close your eyes. Let the hot steam penetrate your face. Take deep, relaxing breaths. After 5 minutes, pat dry. Apply moisturizer. Your skin will have a healthy glow.

Facial Scrubs

Although there are many different types of herbal facial scrubs on the market, they all do basically the same things—they cleanse the skin by removing dirt, excess oil, and dead skin cells. Since most scrubs are slightly abrasive, they can be irritating to very sensitive skin. As a rule, they should not be used more than 2 or 3 times a weekly (and even less often if your skin is dry). There are many wonderful herbal scrubs on the market that include traditional herbs such as apricot, aloe, and almond. Some of the more exotic ones are worth a try. For example, one popular store sells an exfoliating cleanser made out of finely ground Japanese azuki beans. I personally have found it to be excellent. If you want to save money, it's very easy to make your own scrub. A handful of dried almond meal mixed in a little water does the job quite nicely. (Be sure to avoid getting the mixture in your eyes.) Rinse well and apply a moisturizer.

Herbal Facial Mask

A facial mask or peel eliminates the top layers of dead cells and also helps to tighten enlarged pores. It leaves the skin looking smooth and refreshed. There are several fine herbal products on the market, but it's easy enough to make your own mask with herbs that you probably have around the house. Mix 1 teaspoon of peppermint leaves in boiling water. Strain and save the water. To peppermint leaves, mix in 1 tablespoon of dried almond meal and 1 tablespoon of oatmeal. Add a few tablespoons of the water

261

to make a thick paste. Apply to a clean face. Be sure to avoid your eyes. Wait 15 minutes or until mask is dry. Wash off with a warm washcloth. Your face will feel tingling clean. Apply moisturizer.

Quick Facial Mask

Mash a fresh papaya and rub on clean face. Let dry. Wash off with warm water and washcloth.

Terrific Herbal Skin Toner

For a quick pick-me-up, make an herbal skin freshener by mixing liquid witch hazel (you can buy it in any drugstore) with a splash of chamomile tea. When you need to feel (and look) revived, dab a small amount of this mixture on your face with a cotton ball.

Herbs That May Help Prevent Wrinkles

There are several theories of aging that are being given serious consideration these days. (I say theories because we still don't know exactly what triggers the aging process.) One of the more interesting theories concerns the formation of free radicals, destructive forms of oxygen molecules that subvert normal cell function and damage healthy cells. Free radicals are suspected of causing many forms of cancer. They are also believed to accelerate aging.

Antioxidants are substances that can prevent these free radicals from doing their damage. Herbs that contain antioxidants may indirectly help prevent outward signs of aging, such as wrinkles, by stopping free radicals dead in their tracks. These herbs include ginkgo and chaparral. Vitamin E is also a potent antioxidant. We still don't know whether these antioxidants work better if taken orally or rubbed into the skin, or even if they will work at all to help prevent wrinkles. However, I personally feel that anyone who is concerned about wrinkles and other manifestations of aging should consider taking at least one of these antioxidant herbs.

Another way to avoid wrinkles is to stay out of the sun. During the summer, be sure to wear a sunscreen on your face even when you're not officially sunbathing. And although there is no hard evidence to back this claim, many herbalists say that aloe gel can help prevent wrinkles. Considering all the wonderful things that aloe can do for skin, it certainly seems plausible that aloe may indeed help keep skin softer and younger looking.

CHAPTER 10

Aromatherapy

The way to health is to have an aromatic bath and a scented massage every day.

HIPPOCRATES

Whenever I get a whiff of eucalyptus oil, it takes me back to my childhood in Canada. My family would go to a hotel that had a steam bath in the basement, where my father and I would trek periodically to "cleanse our pores" and inhale the fumes emitted from buckets full of fresh eucalyptus leaves floating in hot water. I'll never forget the effect of those eucalyptus leaves—my sinuses would clear, my thoughts would become sharper, and I would leave the steam bath feeling exhilarated.

Many years later, when I learned about aromatherapy, I understood the lure of those steam baths. The power of scent is the guiding principle behind aromatherapy: the use of scented oils to soothe, relax, and heal. In some cases, aromatherapy is also used to treat specific medical problems. Massaged into the skin, certain oils can relieve muscle aches and pains. Some oils are also strongly antiseptic. When an epidemic of plague broke out in ancient Athens, Hippocrates urged the people to burn aromatic plants on the street corners to prevent the plague from spreading. Even in those primitive times, the father of modern medicine somehow knew that the oils emitted by these plants were strong antibiotics that could kill airborne bacteria. Centuries later, researchers in the Soviet Union discovered that eucalyptus oil, a powerful natural antiviral agent, was useful for treating certain strains of influenza.

Today, essential oils are usually used externally: They may be inhaled, rubbed into the skin, or used in the bath. They may also be taken internally (in a diluted form) as medicine, but only under the supervision of a qualified practitioner. (A full-strength essential oil should never be taken orally—it can be very irritating.)

One of the fastest-growing modes of alternative medicine, aromatherapy has been practiced since ancient times. The Egyptians rubbed cumin on their bodies prior to intercourse to promote conception. They also used strong oils in the embalming and mummification process, probably as disinfectants. Ancient Romans wore a garland of roses on the head to cure headaches. Native Americans used the oil of the morning glory to prevent nightmares and prickly ash perfume to promote feelings of love.

The handful of scientific studies that have been done on aromatherapy only reinforce the therapeutic value of essential oils. For example, researchers at Milan University have successfully treated depression and anxiety using aerosol (sprayed) oils. Once inhaled through the nose, the essential oils stimulated the olfactory organs, which are linked to the areas of the brain that control emotions. According to aromatherapists, when these essential oils are rubbed on the skin, they stimulate a reaction on the nerve endings on the skin's surface. This reaction passes through the nerves until it reaches the pituitary or master gland. In turn, through a series of chemical reactions, the pituitary controls whether we feel stressed or relaxed.

Different oils elicit different physical and emotional responses. Some calm us down; some excite us. Some make us happy; some make us reflective. Some enhance our spiritual side; some increase our desire for carnal pleasures.

Essential oils can be purchased at herb shops and health food stores. They are very strong—a little goes a long way. Never inhale from the bottle directly. Rather, mix 1 or 2 drops into a bowl of steaming hot water. Place a towel over your head and around the bowl to catch the steam. If you want to use an essential oil in the bath, place 5 or 6 drops in the warm water. For massage, use 3 or 4 drops of the appropriate scented oil.

The following is a list of commonly used essential oils and the response they are believed to evoke.

1. Apple—Cheers you up
2. Basil—Promotes peace and happiness
3. Bay leaf—Increases psychic awareness
4. Benzoin—Promotes energy
5. Bergamot—Promotes a restful sleep
6. Bergamot mint—Increases energy
7. Black pepper—Increases alertness
8. Broom—Promotes tranquility
9. Calendula—Promotes good health
10. Camphor—Increases energy
11. Caraway—Increases energy
12. Cardomon—Promotes feelings of love and desire for sex
13. Carnation—Increases energy
14. Catnip—Calms you down
15. Cedar—Increases spirituality
16. Celery—Promotes a restful sleep

17. Chamomile—Promotes sleep and tranquility
18. Cinnamon—Increases energy and awareness
19. Clove—Promotes healing
20. Coffee—Enhances the conscious mind
21. Coriander—Improves memory
22. Cumin—Immune booster
23. Cypress—Promotes healing
24. Daffodil—Increases feelings of love
25. Deer tongue—Sexually arousing
26. Dill—Sharpens the conscious mind
27. Eucalyptus—Promotes healing
28. Fennel—Promotes longevity
29. Frankincense—Increases spirituality
30. Gardenia—Promotes feelings of peace and love
31. Garlic—Promotes health, purifies the body
32. Geranium—Promotes happiness
33. Ginger—Increases energy
34. Honeysuckle—Helps weight loss
35. Hops—Promotes sleep
36. Hyacinth—Helps to overcome grief
37. Hyssop—Purifies the body
38. Iris—Increases feelings of love
39. Jasmine—Promotes love, sex, and sleep
40. Juniper—Promotes healing
41. Lavender—Good for health
42. Lemon—Promotes health, healing, and energy
43. Lemon grass—Purifies the body
44. Lemon verbena—Increases feelings of love
45. Lilac—Increases feelings of love
46. Lily—Promotes inner peace
47. Lily of the valley—Improves memory
48. Lime—Increases energy
49. Magnolia—Promotes feelings of love
50. Marjoram—Promotes sleep
51. Mimosa—Promotes psychic dreams
52. Myrrh—Promotes healing

53. Narcissus—Enhances feelings of love
54. Nutmeg—Increases energy
55. Onion—Immune booster
56. Orange—Increases joy and energy
57. Parsley—Protection
58. Pennyroyal—Increases energy
59. Peppermint—Sharpens the conscious mind
60. Pine—Promotes healing
61. Rose—Promotes feelings of love and peace
62. Rosemary—Promotes longevity
63. Rue—Calms you down
64. Saffron—Increases energy
65. Sage—Improves memory
66. Sandalwood—Aphrodisiac and promotes healing
67. Spearmint—Promotes healing
68. Star anise—Increases awareness
69. Sweet pea—Promotes happiness
70. Thyme—Promotes good health
71. Tulip—Purifies the body
72. Vanilla—Promotes sex and love
73. Water lily—Promotes peace and happiness
74. Wood aloe—Increases feelings of love
75. Yarrow—Increases awareness
76. Ylang ylang—Promotes sex and love

Resources

WHERE TO FIND AN HERBALLY AWARE MEDICAL PRACTITIONER

Throughout the *Herb Bible*, I recommend working with a knowledgeable medical practitioner whenever possible. Although it may not be easy to find a doctor who is familiar with natural remedies—or one who is open-minded enough to consider using them—there are places to go for help. The following is a list of organizations that can help you locate medical professionals in your area:

American Holistic Medical Association
2002 Eastlake Avenue East
Seattle, Washington 98102
Tel: 206-322-6842

American Association of Naturopathic Physicians
P.O. Box 20386
Seattle, Washington 98102
Tel: 206-323-7610
Naturopathic physicians are graduates of a four-year postgraduate program in the basic medical sciences. Their training also

includes courses in nutrition and botanical medicine. Although they must pass a national licensing examination, only ten states allow naturopathic physicians to diagnose and treat patients. In other states, a naturopathic physician may work under the supervision of an M.D.

For more information on herbal medicine, write to the following organizations:

The American Botanical Council
P.O. Box 201660
Austin, Texas 78720

The Herb Research Foundation
1007 Pearl Street
Suite 200
Boulder, Colorado 80302
The American Botanical Council and The Herb Research Foundation publish Herbalgram, *an excellent review of the latest developments in botanical medicine. To subscribe, call 800-748-2617.*

A GUIDE TO MAIL-ORDER HERBAL COMPANIES

If you don't live near an herb shop or a health food store, or if you find that some of the herbs mentioned in this book are hard to find, you may need to buy your herbs through a mail-order company. The following is a list of some of the companies in the United States and Canada that offer mail-order service. You can call or write them for a catalogue or product list:

United States

Nature's Herbs
113 North Industrial Park Drive
Orem, Utah 84057
Tel: 801-225-4443

Nature's Way
P.O. Box 4000
Springville, Utah 84883
Tel: 800-9-NATURE

Eclectic Institute
11231 S.E. Market Street
Portland, Oregon 97216
Tel: 800-332-HERB

Solaray
Ogden, Utah 84663

Wakunaga
23501 Madero
Mission Viejo, California 92691
Tel: 800-544-5800

Acta Health Products
1979 East Locust Street
Pasadena, California 91107

Four Seasons Herb Company
17 Buccaneer Street
Marina Del Rey, California 90292
(Specializes in oriental herbs)

Bio-Botanica, Inc.
75 Commerce Drive
Hauppauge, New York 11788
Tel: 516-231-5522

Earthrise Company
P.O. Box 1196
San Rafael, California 94915
Tel: 415-485-0521

Threshold
23 Janesway
Scotts Valley, California 95066
Tel: 408-438-1144

Excel
3280 West Hacienda
Las Vegas, Nevada 89041
Tel: 702-795-7464

Yerba Prima
P.O. Box 5009
Berkeley, California 94705
Tel: 415-632-7477

Canada

Trophic Canada Ltd.
260 Okanagan Avenue East
Penticton, B.C. V2A357
Tel: 604-492-8820

Flora Distributors Ltd.
7400 Fraser Park Drive
Burnaby, B.C. VSJ5B9
Tel: 604-438-1133

Swiss Herbal Remedies
181 Don Park Road
Markham, Ontario L3R1C2
Tel: 416-475-6345

QUEST
1781 West 75th Avenue
Vancouver, B.C. V6P6P2
Tel: 604-261-0611

The Herb Works
P.O. Box 450
Fergus, Ontario N1M1N8
Tel: 519-824-4280

VITA Health
150 Beghin Avenue
Winnipeg, MB R2J3W2
Tel: 204-661-8386

BIO-FORCE
4001 Cote Verth
Montreal, PQ H4R1R5
Tel: 514-335-9393

Bibliography

"Aloe Vera: The Powerful Healing Herb." *The Vitamin Connection:* 37–39, Nov./Dec. 1990.

Austin, Frederick G. "Schistosoma Mansoni Chemoprohylaxis with Dietary Lapachol." *The American Journal of Tropical Medicine and Hygiene:* 412–419. Vol 23, No. 3, 1974.

Blumenthal, Mark. "A Guide to Sedative Herbs." *Health Food Business:* 40–67, June 1990.

——. "Herbal Update." *Whole Foods:* 48, April 1991.

——. "South American Herbs." *Health Foods Business:* 52–53, February 1990.

Boericke, William. *Pocket Manual of Homeopathic Materia Medica.* Phil., PA: Boericke & Runyon, 1927.

"Botanical Field Producing Hearty Growth Areas." *Whole Foods:* 46–98, November 1990.

"Botanicals Generally Recognized as Safe." Herb Research Foundation, Boulder, CO.

Botanical Research Summaries, Eclectic Dispensatory of Botanical Therapeutics. Eclectic Institute, Portland, OR.

Briggs, Colin J. "Evening Primrose: La Belle de Nuit, The King's Cureall." *Canadian Pharmacy Journal* 119 (5): 249–252, 54, May 1986.

Brody, Jane E. "Personal Health: A note of caution in exploring the world of medicinal herbs: It's a jungle out there." *The New York Times:* Feb. 15, 1990.

————. "Fortified Foods Could Fight Off Cancer." *The New York Times:* February 19, 1991.

Brown, Donald. "Botanical Medicine in America: The Medical Connection." *Let's Live:* 50–52, February 1990.

"Capsules." (The Pacific Yew Tree.) *Pharmacy West:* 30, January 1991.

Carter, James P. "Gamma-Linolenic Acid as a Nutrient." *Food Technology* 42 (6): 72, 74–75, 78–79, 81–82, June 1988.

Castleman, Michael. "Friend or Foe?" (Comfrey) *The Herb Quarterly* 44: 18–23, Winter 1989.

————. "An Herbal Remedy for Migraines." *The Herb Quarterly* 43: 8–11, Fall 1989.

Chihal, Jane H. "Premenstrual Syndrome: An Update for the Clinician." *Obstetrics and Gynecology Clinics of North America* 17 (2): 457–479, June 1990.

Colbin, Annemarie. *Food and Healing.* New York: Ballantine Books. 1986.

Crellin, John K., and Philpott, Jane. *Herbal Medicine Past and Present, Volume 2. A Reference Guide to Medicinal Plants.* Durham: Duke University Press, 1990.

Culpeper, Nicholas. *Culpeper's Complete Herbal.* London: W. Foulsham & Co., Ltd.

Dobelis, I., and Ferguson, G. *Reader's Digest Magic and Medicine of Plants*. Pleasantville, NY: Reader's Digest Books, 1986.

Farnsworth, Norman R., Akerele, O., et al. "Medicinal Plants in Therapy." *Bulletin of the World Health Organization:* 63 (6) 965-981, 1985.

Fox, Timothy R. "Aloe Vera: Revered, Mysterious Healer." *Health Foods Business:* 45–46, December 1990.

Gabriel, Ingrid. *Herb Identifier and Handbook*. New York: Sterling Publishing Company, 1979.

"Garlic Folk and Fact." *Whole Foods:* 75, January 1991.

Grandinetti, Deborah. *Prevention:* 48–50, December 1988.

Hassam, A. G. "The Role of Evening Primrose Oil in Nutrition and Disease." *The Role of Fats in Human Nutrition*. Chichester, England: Ellis Horwood, 1985.

Hausman, Patricia, and Hurley, Judith Benn. *The Healing Foods: The Ultimate Authority on the Curative Power of Nutrition*. Emmaus, PA: Rodale Press, 1989.

Hepinstal, S., et al. "Extracts of feverfew inhibit granule secretion in blood platelets and polymorphonuclear leucocytes." *The Lancet:* 1071–1073, May 11, 1985.

————, White, Anne, Williamson, L., et al. "Extracts of Feverfew Inhibit Granule Secretion in Blood Platelets and Polymorphonuclear Leucocytes." *The Lancet:* 1071–1073, May 11, 1985.

"Herb: Just Another 4-Letter Word for Drug." *Longevity:* 51–55, April 1991.

"Herbs for Healthy Skin and Hair." *Whole Foods:* 84, October 1990.

"Origins of Nutrition and Diabetes." *Nutrition Today:* 13–18, Jan./Feb. 1991.

Hobbs, Christopher. "The Chaste Tree: Vitex agnus castus." *Pharmacy in History* 33 (1): 19–22, 1991.

Holmes, Peter. *The Energetics of Western Herbs: Integrating Western and Oriental Herbal Medicine Traditions.* Vol. 1. Boulder, CO: Artemis Press, 1989.

Horrobin, David F., and Manku, Mehar S. "Clinical Biochemistry of Essential Fatty Acids." *Omega–6 Essential Fatty Acids: Pathophysiology and Roles in Clinical Medicine.* Alan R. Liss, Inc: 21–53.

Kail, Konrad. "Natural Stimulants." *Health Foods Business:* 51–52, January 1991.

Kloss, Jethro. *Back to Eden.* Loma Linda, CA: Back to Eden Publishing Company, 1936.

Kronick, Jeff. "New Ways of Looking at Herbs for Americans." *Whole Foods:* 54–56, February 1990.

"Oil of Evening Primrose." *Lawrence Review of Natural Products.* March 1989.

Leung, Albert Y. "The Proper Use of Herbs." *Whole Foods:* 81–83, November 1990.

Leung, Albert Y. "The Herbal News." 2: Fall 1990.

Longcope, Christopher. "Relationships of Estrogen to Breast Cancer, of Diet to Breast Cancer, and of Diet to Estradiol Metabolism." *Journal of the National Cancer Institute* 82 (11), June 6, 1990.

Leyel, C. F. *Herbal Delights.* New York: Gramercy Publishing Company, 1938.

Lucas, Richard. *Common and Uncommon Uses of Herbs for Healthful Living*. West Nyack, NY: Parker Publishing Company, Inc., 1969.

Lust, John. *The Herb Book*. New York: Bantam Books, 1974.

Mabley, Richard. *The New Age Herbalist*. London: Gaia Books, 1988.

Mars, Brigette. "Herbs to Know About During Pregnancy." *Let's Live*: 74–75, February 1991.

McCaleb, Rob. "What's New With Ginseng?" Herb Research Foundation, December 18, 1990.

Michnovicz, Jon, and Bradlow, H. Leon. "Induction of Estradiol Metabolism by Dietary Indole-3-carbinol in Humans. *Journal of the National Cancer Institute* 82 (11), June 6, 1990.

Mindell, Earl. *Vitamin Bible*. New York: Warner Books, 1985.

Mowry, Daniel B. *Guaranteed Potency Herbs: Next Generation Herbal Medicine*. New Canaan, CT: Keats Publishing Company, 1990.

Murphy, J. J., Hepinstall, S., and Mitchell, J. R. A. "Randomized Double-Blind Placebo Controlled Trial of Feverfew in Migraine Prevention." *The Lancet*: 189–192. July 23, 1988.

Murty, N. Anjneya, and Pandey, D. P. *Ayurvedic Cure for Common Diseases*. New Delhi: Orient Paperbacks, 1982.

Passwater, Richard A. "Antioxidant Nutrients and Heart Disease." *Whole Foods*: 49–52.

Peterson, Nicola. *Culpeper Guides: Herbs and Health*. London: Webb & Bower, 1989.

Rose, Jeanne. *Modern Herbal*. New York: Perigee Books, 1987.

Ryman, Daniele. *The Aromatherapy Handbook*. Essex, England: The C. W. Daniel Company, Ltd., 1989.

Santillo, Humbart. *Natural Healing with Herbs*. Prescott Valley, AZ: Hohm Press, 1984.

Shewell-Cooper, W. E. *Plants, Flowers and Herbs of the Bible*. New Canaan, CT: Keats Publishing, 1977.

Shibata, Shoji, Tanaka Osamu, et al. "Chemistry and Pharmacology of Panax." *Economic and Medicinal Plant Research* 1:218–284. London: Academic Press Inc., 1985.

Stanway, Andrew. *The Natural Family Doctor: The Comprehensive Self-Help Guide to Health and Natural Medicine*. London: Gaia Books Ltd., 1987.

Stolzenburg, William. "Garlic Medicine: Cures in Cloves?" *Science News:* 157, Sept. 8, 1990.

Swenson A. Allen. *Your Biblical Garden: Plants of the Bible and How to Grow Them*. Garden City, NY: Doubleday and Co., 1981.

Teeguarden, Ron. *Chinese Herbal Tonics*. Tokyo: Japan Publications, 1984.

"The Top Ten Herbs of the '90s." *Health Food Business:* 46–83, October 1989.

Tisserand, Robert. *Aromatherapy: To Heal and Tend the Body*. Santa Fe: Lotus Press, 1988.

New Tobe, John H. Tobe. *Proven Herbal Remedies*. Ontario, Canada: Provoker Press, 1969.

Tyler, Varro E. "Plant Drugs in the 21st Century." *Economic Botany* 40 (3): 279–288, 1986.

"Up & Coming Herbs: A Look Toward the Herbal Horizon." *Whole Foods:* 24–26, April 1991.

"Vulnerable Yew Tree Yields Cancer Treatment." *National Geographic*, April 1991.

Wagner, H., Kikino, Hiroshi, and Farnsworth, Norman, R. "Siberian Ginseng (Eleutherococcus senticosus): Current Status as an Adaptogen." *Economic and Medicinal Plant Research*, 1:156–215. London: Academic Press, 1985.

Ward, Harold. *Herbal Manual*. London: The C.W. Daniel Company Ltd., 1936.

Weed, Susan S. *Wise Woman Herbal Childbearing Year*. Woodstock, NY: Ash Tree Publishing, 1986.

Weil, Andrew. "A New Look at Botanical Medicine." *Whole Earth Review* 64, Fall 1989.

Weiner, Michael. *Herbs and Immunity*. San Rafael, CA: Quantum Books, 1990.

———. "Native American Herbs: A New Look at a National Resource." *Health Foods Business*: 62–66, March 1991.

———. "Herbs and Energy." *The Herbal Healthline*. 1 (3): 1–14.

———. *Weiner's Herbal*. Mill Valley, CA: Quantum Books, 1990.

Williams III, Gurney. "$5 Million a Year for Herbs . . . and Still Counting." *Longevity*: 56–64, April 1991.

"Women Healers on Women's Health." *EastWest: The Journal of Natural Health & Living*, November 1990.

Zand, Janet. "Herbal Programs for Women's Health." *Health Foods Business*: 40–41, January 1991.

In addition, *Herbalgram*, a newsletter which has been published by the Herb Research Foundation since 1983, proved to be an invaluable resource.

Index

Abdominal pain, anise, 41
Acetaminophen, 14
Aerosol oils, 266
Aging
  chaparral and, 72
  fo-ti and, 96
  ginkgo and, 103
  and herbs, 249–250
Alfalfa, 35–36, 192
Allantoin, 74
Allergies
  chamomile and, 71
  herbs for, 170, 218
  psyllium and, 150
  see also Hayfever
Allium, uses of, 248
Almond, 36–37, 192
Aloe vera, 37–39, 192
Alzheimer's disease, ginkgo
  and, 103

Amalaki, 209
Amenorrhea, elecampane
  and, 179
American gingseng, 108–109
Anemia
  asparagus and, 46
  dandelion and, 79
  dong quai and, 82
  herbs for, 236
Angelica, 39–41
Animals, and herbs, 28
Anise, 41–42
Antiemetic, cloves, 74
Antihistamine, reishi mushroom, 170
Anti-inflammatories
  goldenseal, 112
  white willow bark, 166
  witch hazel, 185
  yucca, 167

Antiparasitics
  black walnut, 54
  chaparral, 72
Antiseptics
  black walnut, 54
  eucalyptus, 88
  myrrh, 133
  onion, 139
Antispasmodics
  angelica, 40
  peppermint, 147
Anxiety
  evening primrose and, 90
  lavender and, 180
  St. John's Wort and, 154
Aphrodisiacs
  artichoke, 45
  cloves, 74
  damiana, 78
  ginseng, 107
  jasmine, 122
  for women, 236
Appetite
  alfalfa and, 35
  blessed thistle and, 55
  caraway and, 64
  cayenne and, 62
  celery and, 69
  dill and, 81
  fennel and, 92
  hyssop and, 121
  lady's mantle and, 125
  see also Indigestion
Apple, 42–43
Arnica, 43–44
Aromatherapy, 265–269
Arthritis
  asparagus and, 46
  burdock and, 58
  butcher's broom and, 59
  devil's claw and, 80
  eucalyptus and, 88

herbs for, 222–223
  licorice and, 127
  sarsaparilla and, 157
  turmeric and, 163
  white willow bark and,
    166
  yucca and, 167
Artichoke, 44–45
  heart and, 247
  and the liver, 251
Ashwagandha, 209
Asparagus, 45–46
Aspirin, 12
  meadowsweet and, 181
  white willow bark and,
    166
Asthma, parsley and, 142
Astragalus, 47–48, 197
  immune system and, 250
Astringent, bayberry bark,
  50
Athlete's foot, herbs for,
  226
Autoimmune problems, al-
  falfa and, 36
Ayurveda, 113, 207–210
  practice of, 207

Backache
  burdock and, 58
  chamomile and, 70
  mustard and, 182
Ba Dan Xing Ren, 192
Baldness, 240–241
Basil, 49, 193
Bayberry bark, 49–51
Bean curd, 193
Bearberry. See Uva ursi
Bible
  aloe vera and, 37
  and herbs, 186–187
  myrrh and, 133

Bilberry, 51–52
    and vision, 251
Bile, milk thistle and, 131
Bioflavinoids, 253
Black cohosh, 52–53
Black walnut, 53–54
Bladder
    infections of, alfalfa and,
        35
    Native American remedies
        for, 212
Bleeding
    blessed thistle and, 55
    lady's mantle and, 125
Blessed thistle, 54–55
Bloating. See Diuretics
Blood clotting
    reishi mushroom and, 170
    turmeric and, 162
Blood pressure
    dandelion and, 79
    dong quai and, 82
    garlic and, 98
    licorice and, 127
    Siberian ginseng and, 110
Blood sugar
    apple and, 43
    dandelion and, 79
    fenugreek and, 93
    nettle and, 135
    pau d'arco and, 145
Bones, horsetail and, 120
Boneset, 55–56
Borage, 176
Bowel functions
    apple and, 43
    basil and, 49
    black walnut and, 54
Brahmi, 209
Break bone fever, 56
Breast-feeding, garlic and,
    99

Breath fresheners, herbs for,
    224
Bronchitis
    catnip and, 68
    mullein and, 132
Buchu, 56–57
    uva ursi and, 56
Buckthorn. See Cascara
    sagrada
Bulimia, ipecac and, 204
Buplerum, 197
Burdock, 57–58
Burns
    aloe vera and, 38
    calendula and, 60
    ginger and, 101
    herbs for, 221–222
Butcher's broom, 59–60

Calendula, 60–61
Cancer
    American ginseng and,
        109
    astragalus and, 47
    carrots and, 65
    chaparral and, 72
    foods and, 246
    fo-ti and, 96
    garlic and, 99
    ginkgo and, 103
    ginseng and, 107
    and herbs, 34
    licorice and, 127
    onion and, 139
    ovarian, herbs for, 236–
        237
    preventative herbs and,
        248–249
    red clover and, 153
    research into, 245
    shiitake mushrooms and,
        159

Capsicum. *See* Cayenne
Caraway, 63–64
Cardamom, 177
Carotene, 65
Carrot, 65–66
    and cancer, 248
Cascara sagrada, 66–67
Catnip, 67–68
Cavities, licorice and, 127
Cayenne, 61–62, 203
    circulation and, 249
    heart and, 247
Celery, 68–69
Chafed nipples, comfrey
    and, 76
Ch'ai Hu, 197
Chamomile, 69–71
Chaparral, 71–72
    and aging, 249
Chaste tree, 169
Chemotherapy, 30
    astragalus and, 47
    see also Cancer
Chewing gum, 213
Chicken soup, 217
Chickweed, 177
Childbirth
    black cohosh and, 53
    gotu kola and, 114
    herbs for, 235
    motherwort and, 181
    raspberry leaves and,
        151
    see also Episiotomy; Preg-
        nancy
Children, caraway and, 64
Chills, angelica and, 40
Chinese herbal tradition,
    189–202
Chives, 73–74
Cholesterol
    almond and, 37

American ginseng and, 109
apple and, 43
artichoke and, 45
carrots and, 65
cucumber and, 178
evening primrose and, 90
ginseng and, 107
oat fiber and, 136
olive and, 138
reishi mushroom and, 170
shiitake mushroom and,
    159
Siberian ginseng and, 110
Chrysanthemum, 193–194
Circulation
    butcher's broom and, 59
    ginkgo and, 103
    gotu kola and, 114
    hawthorne berries and,
        115
    herbs for, 232, 249
Cleansers, for skin, almond,
    37
Cloves, 74
Club moss, 178
Colds
    cayenne and, 62
    echinacea and, 84
    elder and, 85
    eucalyptus and, 88
    ginger and, 101
    goldenseal and, 112
    herbs for, 215–217
    horehound and, 117
    marshmallow and, 130
    myrrh and, 134
    Native American medicine
        for, 211
    onion and, 139
    pennyroyal and, 146
    Siberian ginseng and, 110
    see also Congestion

Colic
  lemon balm and, 176
  onion and, 140
Colitis, marshmallow and,
  130
Comfrey, 21, 74–76
Concentration, ginkgo and,
  103
Congestion
  anise and, 42
  bayberry bark and, 50
  gotu kola and, 114
  Iceland moss and, 179
  licorice and, 127
  mullein and, 132
  parsley and, 142
  yerba santa and, 167
Constipation
  alfalfa and, 35
  apple and, 43
  cucumber and, 178
  goldenseal and, 112
  herbs for, 220
  olive and, 138
Cough
  arnica and, 44
  black cohosh and, 53
  herbs for, 215–217
  pennyroyal and, 146
Crabs, thyme and, 184
Cramps
  herbs for, 220
  sage and, 184
  St. John's Wort and, 155
Cranberry, 76–78
  juice, 77–78
Cucumber, 178
Culpeper, Nicholas, 30,
  31
Culpepers, herbal shop,
  31
Cynara, 45

Cystitis
  alfalfa and, 35
  uva ursi and, 163

Damiana, 78
Dandelion, 79–80, 194
  history of, 80
  and the liver, 251
Dang Shen, 201
Da T'sao, 199
Decongestant, ephedra, 87
Deer antler. See Lu rong
De Materia Medica (Dio-
  scorides), 29
Deodorants, and herbs,
  224
Devil's claw, 80–81
Diarrhea
  apple and, 43
  carrots and, 66
  catnip and, 68
  chaparral and, 72
  herbs for, 220
  horseradish and, 119
  lungwort and, 128
Digestion
  anise and, 41
  basil and, 49
  caraway and, 63
  celery and, 69
  chamomile and, 70
  chives and, 73
  dandelion and, 79
  elecampane and, 179
  fennel and, 92
  garlic and, 99
  juniper berries and, 123
  papaya and, 141
  parsley and, 142
  pau d'arco and, 145
  peppermint and, 148
  pleurisy root and, 149

Digestion (*cont.*)
 sage and, 184
 see also Gas; Indigestion
Digitalis, 12
Dill, 81
Dioscorides, 29
Disease
 resistance to, astragalus
  and, 47
 treatment of, 18
Disinfectant, thyme, 184
Diuretics, 230
 alfalfa, 35
 artichoke, 45
 asparagus, 46
 astragalus, 47
 buchu, 57
 burdock, 58
 celery, 69
 chaparral, 72
 cucumber, 178
 dandelion, 79
 horehound, 117
 juniper berries, 123
 kava kava, 124
 meadowsweet, 181
 sarsaparilla, 156
 types of herbs, 220
 uva ursi, 163
 Wild Oregon grape, 185
Dizziness
 herbs for, 223–224
 rosemary and, 183
Doctrine of Signatures, 129
Dong quai, 82–83, 198
Don Sen, 198
Dosage, 21, 27–28
Dou Fu (tofu), 193
Driving, passionflower and,
 144
Drugs, and herb use, 18
Drugstores, 16

Earaches, herbs for, 224
Earl Mindell's Vitamin Bible,
 16
Ebers, Georg, 22
Echinacea, 83–85
 freeze drying, 85
 immune system and,
  250
Eczema
 chickweed and, 177
 goldenseal and, 112
Edema, butcher's broom
 and, 59–60
Elder, 85–86
 cooking, 86
Elecampane, 179
Endurance, 242–243
 American ginseng and,
  109
 ginseng and, 107
 sarsaparilla and, 157
*English Physician Enlarged,
 The* (Culpeper), 30, 31
Enteritis, marshmallow and,
 130
Ephedra, 87–88, 198–199
Ephedrine, 12
Episiotomy, herbs for, 233–
 234
Essential oils, 266
 commonly used, 267–269
Eucalyptus, 88–89
 and aromatherapy, 265
Evening primrose, 89–90
Expectorant
 boneset, 56
 caraway, 64
 eucalyptus, 88
 fennel, 92
 fenugreek, 93
 horehound, 117
 horseradish, 119

hyssop, 121
Iceland moss, 179
lungwort, 128
marshmallow, 130
mustard, 182
onion, 139
red clover, 153
saw palmetto, 158
thyme, 184
yerba santa, 167
Eyebright, 91–92
Eye care, and herbs, 259
Eye problems
eyebright and, 91
Native American
medicine for, 212
Eyesight
bilberry and, 51
carrots and, 65

Facial
herbal, 260–261
mask, 261–262
scrubs, 261
toner for, 262
Fang-feng, 201
Fan Jia, 196
Fan Mu Gua, 196
Fatigue, suma and, 161
Female herbs
dong quai, 82
see also Menopause; Men-
struation; Pregnancy
Fennel, 92–93
Fenugreek, 93–94
Fever
blessed thistle and, 55
boneset and, 56
calendula and, 60
herbs for, 218
horse chestnut and,
118

Fever blisters, raspberry
leaves and, 151
Feverfew, 94–96
Fleming, Sir Alexander, 22
Flu
boneset and, 56
echinacea and, 84
herbs for, 215–217
Folic acid deficiency, asparagus and, 46
Fo-ti, 96–97, 199
and aging, 249
Foxglove, 21
heart and, 48
Fungal infections
black walnut and, 54
pau d'arco and, 145

Gallbladder
dandelion and, 79
turmeric and, 163
Gamma linolenic acid, 89
Gan Cao, 195–196
Gan Jiang, 195
Garlic, 21, 97–100, 194
circulation and, 249
heart and, 247
immune system and, 250
Gas
anise and, 41
basil and, 49
caraway and, 63
catnip and, 68
dill and, 81
garlic and, 99
herbs for, 218–219
hyssop and, 121
lemon balm and, 176
oat fiber and, 136
peppermint and, 147
sage and, 184
valerian and, 165

Gastrointestinal
  infections, psyllium and,
    150
Gastrointestinal stress, mullein and, 131
Gay Gee, 199–200
Gerard, John, 30
Gin, juniper berries and,
    123
Ginger, 100–102, 195
Ginkgo, 102–104
  and aging, 249–250
  and circulation, 249
Ginseng, 104–108, 195
  heart and, 246
Goldenseal, 111–113
Gotu kola, 113–115
Gout
  celery and, 69
  juniper berries and, 123
Grooming products, 255
Guarana, 203
Guduchi, 210
Gum disease
  goldenseal and, 112
  myrrh and, 133

Hahnemann, Samuel, 30
Hair
  color, and herbs, 257–258
  conditioning herbs, 256–
    257
  growth of, and herbs, 258
  horsetail and, 120
  olive and, 138
  and shampoo residue,
    257–258
Hamlet, and herbs, 183
Hands, chapped, herbs for,
    260
Hawthorne berries, 115–
  116

Hayfever
  eyebright and, 92
  nettle and, 135
Headaches
  ephedra and, 87
  herbs for, 223
  passionflower and, 143
  rosemary and, 183
Health food stores, 16
Heart
  disease, psyllium and, 150
  fo-ti and, 96
  hawthorne berries and, 115
  health of, 246–248
  onion and, 139
Hemorrhoids
  bayberry bark and, 50
  butcher's broom and, 59
  cayenne and, 63
  ginkgo and, 103
  herbs for, 232–233
  horse chestnut and, 118
  oat fiber and, 136
  witch hazel and, 185
Hepatitis
  milk thistle and, 131
  Wild Oregon grape and,
    185
Herbalism
  decline of, 13
  history of, 28–31
  practitioners of, 245, 271–
    272
*Herball or General Historie of
  Plantes, The* (Gerard),
    30
Herbal remedies, 215
  interest in, 14
  timing of, 28
Herbal tea
  making of, 171
  types of, 170–173

Herbs
  availability of, 23
  buying of, 22–23
  Chinese, 29, 191
  and the church, 29
  consumers and, 26
  definition of, 19
  and the five tastes, 207
  freeze-dried, 23
  function of, 21
  guides for, 16
  guides to, 29
  hazards of, 21–22, 34
    see also particular herbs
  'Hot Hundred', 33–173
    use of, 34
  packaging methods,
    24–26
  and patents, 13–14
  quality of, 26
  shelf life, 26
  shops, 23
  standardization of, 23
  use of, 15, 21
  for women, 227–237
  women's role in history
    of, 227
Herpes zoster. See Shingles
Hippocrates, 27, 29, 265
Hops, 116
Horehound, 117
Hormone balancer, chaste
  tree, 169
Hormone production, asparagus and, 46
Horse chestnut, 117–118
Horseradish, 118–120
Horsetail, 120–121
Ho Shou, 199
Huang Chi, 197
Hu Suan, 194
Hyssop, 121–122

Iceland moss, 179–180
Immune system
  echinacea and, 84
  and herbs, 250
  osha and, 169
  shiitake mushrooms and,
    159
Impotency, 242
Indigestion
  carrots and, 66
  catnip and, 68
  cayenne and, 62
  dill and, 81
  goldenseal and, 112
  herbs for, 218–219
  hops and, 116
  oat fiber and, 136
  papaya and, 141
  see also Colic
Indoles, uses of, 248
Infection
  chaparral and, 72
  garlic and, 98
Inflammation
  cayenne and, 62
  chaparral and, 72
Insect bites, aloe vera and,
  38
Insect repellant, pennyroyal,
  147
Insomnia
  lemon balm and, 176
  peppermint and, 148
  Siberian ginseng and,
    111
  skullcap and, 160
  valerian and, 165
Ipecac, 203–204
Iron, nettle and, 135
Iron deficiency, chives and,
  73
Itching, herbs for, 222

Jasmine, 122
Jaundice, Wild Oregon
grape and, 185
Jie Eng, 200
Joint pain
arnica and, 44
fennel and, 92
mustard and, 182
see also Rheumatism
Jujube date. See Da t'sao
Juniper berries, 123

Kava kava, 124
Keetwuah, Cherokee healer,
213
Kidneys
asparagus and, 46
buchu and, 57
myrrh and, 134
Native American medicine
for, 212
Ko Ken, 200

Lady's mantle, 125–126
Latin Pharmacopeia, 31
Lavender, 180
Laxatives
aloe vera, 38
boneset, 56
cascara sagrada, 67
damiana, 78
Native American, 212
psyllium, 150
Lemon balm, 175–176
Leyel, C.F., 31
Lice
angelica and, 40
herbs for, 222
thyme and, 184
Licorice, 21, 126–127, 195–
196
and cancer, 248

Lifestyle
effects of, 255
health of, 17
herbs and, 33
Light sensitivity, St. John's
Wort and, 155
Liver
artichoke and, 45
blessed thistle and, 55
dandelion and, 79
herbs for, 250–251
milk thistle and, 131
turmeric and, 162
Wild Oregon grape and,
185
Lu Hui, 192
Lungwort, 128
Luole, 193
Lu Rong, 197
Lycii. See Gay gee

Mad dog weed. See Skullcap
Ma Huang, 198
Mail-order companies, for
herbs, 272–275
Mandrakes, 186
Marijuana, 144
Marshmallow, 129–130
Mate, 204
Meadowsweet, 180–181
Medications, hazards of,
14–15
Medicine
and aromatherapy, 266
herbal. See Herbalism
preventative, 15
Memory, gotu kola and, 114
Men, herbs for, 239–244
Menopause
dong quai and, 82
ginseng and, 107
herbs for, 228–229

Menstruation
  blessed thistle and, 55
  calendula and, 60
  celery and, 69
  dong quai and, 82
  herbs for, 230–231
  irregularity of, herbs for,
    234
  lady's mantle and, 125
  nettle and, 135
  parsley and, 142
  pennyroyal and, 146
  raspberry leaves and, 151
  see also PMS
Mi Die Xiang, 196
Migraine headaches
  feverfew and, 95
  peppermint and, 148
Milk production
  anise and, 42
  caraway and, 64
  dill and, 81
Milk thistle, 130–131
  and the liver, 250
Moisturizers
  almond, 37
  aloe vera, 38
  herbs for, 221
Mormon tea. See Ephedra
Morning sickness
  ginger and, 101
  herbs for, 234–235
Motherwort, 181
Motion sickness
  ginger and, 102
  herbs for, 223–224
Mouth sores
  feverfew and, 96
  myrrh and, 133
Mouthwash, herbs for, 221
Mullein, 132–133
Muria puama, 204–205

Muscles
  arnica and, 44
  black cohosh and, 53
  herbs for, 222–223
  passionflower and, 143
Muscle strains, 243–244
Muscle tension
  skullcap and, 160
  valerian and, 165
Mushrooms. See Reishi
    mushroom; Shiitake
    mushroom
Mustard, 182
Muxu, 192
Myopia, bilberry and, 51
Myrrh, 133–134
  goldenseal and, 112

Nails
  and herbs, 259
  horsetail and, 120
Names of herbs, 20
Native American herb tradi-
    tion, 30, 210–213
Nausea
  anise and, 41
  basil and, 49
  caraway and, 63
  herbs for, 219
Nephritis, uva ursi and, 163
Nervous tension
  lemon balm and, 176
  rosemary and, 183
  skullcap and, 160
  see also Relaxants
Nettle, 134–135
Neuralgia
  black cohosh and, 53
  white willow bark and,
    166
Night blindness, bilberry
    and, 51

North American Indians.
  See Native American herb
    tradition
Nursing, herbs for, 235
Nutrition
  alfalfa and, 35
  herbal sources, 253

Oat bran, 136–137
  heart and, 247
Oil, horsetail and, 120
Olfactory organs, 266
Olive, 137–138
Olive oil, heart and, 247
Oncologists, 34
Onion, 138–140
Osha, 168–169
Osteoporosis, 237
Ovarian cancer. *See* Cancer

Pain reliever
  hops, 116
  white willow bark, 166
Pai Shu, 200
Papaya, 140–141, 196
Parasitic infection, pau
    d'arco and, 145
Parsley, 142–143
Passionflower, 143–144
Pau d'arco, 144–145, 205
Pectin, 42
Penicillin, 13, 22
Pennyroyal, 146–147
Pepper, hot, 196
Peppermint, 147–148
Pharmaceutical companies,
  14
Pharmacognosy, 11–12
Pharmacy, herbal, 20
Pharmacy school, 11
Phlebitis, gotu kola and,
  114

Phlegm
  angelica and, 40
  pleurisy root and, 149
  red clover and, 153
  yerba santa and, 167
Photosynthesis, 19
Physicians, homeopathic, 30
Planta Medica, 84
Plants, components of, 20
Platycodon, 200
Pleurisy root, 148–149
PMS
  borage and, 176
  dong quai and, 82
  evening primrose and, 90
  herbs for 229–230
  motherwort and, 181
  pennyroyal and, 146
Poisoning, nettle and, 135
Pregnancy
  angelica and, 41
  black cohosh and, 53
  blessed thistle and, 55
  calendula and, 61
  celery and, 69
  devil's claw and, 81
  dong quai and, 83
  elecampane and, 179
  gotu kola and, 115
  and herbs, 22, 34
  juniper berries and, 123
  motherwort and, 181
  myrrh and, 134
  Native American birth
    control herbs, 213
  olive and, 138
  parsley and, 143
  pennyroyal and, 147
  raspberry leaves and, 152
  see also Childbirth
Premenstrual syndrome. *See*
  PMS

Primrose oil, and heart, 246
Prostate problems, 239–240
  saw palmetto and, 158
Pseudoephedrine, 12
Psyllium, 149–151
  heart and, 247
Pueraria, 200
Pu Gong Ying, 194
Pyrroliziidine alkaloids, 75

Quinidine, 12
Quinine, 12

Rainforests, and herbs, 208
Raspberry leaves, 151–152
Red clover, 152–153
Rehmannia, 200
Reishi mushroom, 170
  immune system and,
    250
Relaxants
  black cohosh, 52
  boneset, 56
  catnip, 68
  chamomile, 70
  gotu kola, 114
  hops, 116
  jasmine, 122
  kava kava, 124
  marshmallow, 130
  oat fiber, 136
  passionflower, 143
  red clover, 153
  St. John's Wort, 154
  valerian, 165
Ren Shen, 195
Reserpine, 12
Respiratory tract infections
  elecampane and, 179
  see also Colds; Congestion
Restless leg syndrome,
  herbs for, 232

Rheumatism
  alfalfa and, 35, 36
  angelica and, 40
  apple and, 43
  asparagus and, 46
  black cohosh and, 52
  burdock and, 58
  butcher's broom and, 59
  celery and, 69
  chamomile and, 70
  club moss and, 178
  devil's claw and, 80
  eucalyptus and, 88
  herbs for, 222–223
  horseradish and, 119
  Native American medicine
    for, 212
  sarsaparilla and, 157
  white willow bark and,
    166
  yucca and, 167
Rosemary, 182–183, 196–197

Saffron, 111
Sage, 183–184
St. John's Wort, 154–155
Salvia, 201
Sarsaparilla, 155–157, 205
Saw palmetto, 157–158
Scabies, thyme and, 184
Schizandra chiensis, 201
Schizandra fructus, 201
Self-diagnosis, 18
Sexual organs, saw palmetto
  and, 158
Sexual problems, 242
  see also Aphrodisiacs
Shampoo, 213
Shanka puspi, 210
Shen Nong Ben Cao Jing, 190
Shennong Herbal, 104, 113,
  126

Shiitake mushroom, 158–159
  and cancer, 249
  immune system and, 250
Shingles, calendula and, 60
Siberian ginseng, 110–111
Sileris, 201
Skin
  broken, arnica and, 44
  cleansers, almond, 37
  dry, herbs for, 259–260
  evening primrose and, 90
  herbal care, 259–263
  witch hazel and, 185
  see also Moisturizers
Skin irritation
  aloe vera and, 38
  arnica and, 44
  burdock and, 58
  calendula and, 60
  chamomile and, 70
  chickweed and, 177
  comfrey and, 76
  cucumber and, 178
  elder and, 85
  fenugreek and, 93
  from shaving, 244
  goldenseal and, 112
  herbs for, 222, 224
  mustard and, 182
  olive and, 138
  red clover and, 153
Skin wounds
  comfrey and, 76
  echinacea and, 84
  St. John's Wort and, 155
Skullcap, 159–160
Sleep
  and herbs, 224–225
  kava kava and, 24
  see also Insomnia
Slippery elm bark, 160–161
Society of Herbalists, 31

Sok-day-sang-day, 200
Sore throat
  fenugreek and, 93
  herbs for, 217
  hyssop and, 121
  licorice and, 127
  lungwort and, 128
  Native American medicine
    for, 212
  raspberry leaves and, 151
  slippery elm bark and,
    161
  thyme and, 184
South American herbal tra-
    dition, 202–207
Squaw tea. See Ephedra
Stevia, 206
Stimulants
  American ginseng, 109
  astragalus, 47
  bayberry, bark, 50
  buchu, 57
  cardamom, 177
  cayenne, 62
  ephedra, 87
  ginseng, 107
  and herbs, 225
  Siberian ginseng, 110
  suma, 161
Stomach
  anise and, 41
  ginger and, 101
  lavender and, 180
  lemon balm and, 176
  myrrh and, 133
  see also Appetite; Colic;
    Digestion; Gas; Indiges-
    tion
Stress
  American ginseng and, 109
  ginseng and, 107
  herbs for, 225

Siberian ginseng and, 110
valerian and, 165
Suma, 161–162, 206
Sunburn
chamomile and, 70
herbs for, 221
Sweating
horehound and, 117
sage and, 183
Swelling, in feet, butcher's
broom and, 60

Tang Kuei, 198
Tang Shen, 198
Thyme, 184
Tinnitus, ginkgo and, 103
Tofu. See Dou fu
Tooth pain
cloves and, 74
herbs for, 221
Native American medicine
for, 213
Traditional herbs, 175–187
Turmeric, 162–163
and circulation, 249
and the liver, 251

Ulcers
calendula and, 60
comfrey and, 76
goldenseal and, 112
licorice and, 127
marshmallow and, 130
Unsaturated fatty acids,
253
Urinary problems, sarsaparilla and, 156
Urinary tract infections
buchu and, 57
cranberry and, 77
juniper berries and, 123
licorice and, 127

U.S. Pharmacopeia, 12, 76,
156, 179
Uterine cramping, St. John's
Wort and, 155
Uva ursi, 163–164
buchu and, 56

Vacha, 210
Vaginal infections
goldenseal and, 112
lady's mantle and, 125
nettle and, 135
Vagotonic, horse chestnut
and, 118
Valerian, 164–165
Varicose veins
bayberry bark and, 50
herbs for, 232–233
horse chestnut and, 118
witch hazel and, 185
Vertigo, ginkgo and, 103
Vinblastine, 13
Vincritisine, 13
Viral infections
echinacea and, 84
St. John's Wort and, 155
Vision, and herbs, 251
Vitamin B, oat fiber and,
136
Vitamins, herbal sources,
252
Vitex. See Chaste tree
Vomiting
cloves and, 74
herbs for, 219

Warts, onion and, 139
Water retention. See Diuret-
ics
White willow bark, 165–166
Wild Mexican yam, 206–207
Wild Oregon grape, 185

Wisconsin, ginseng and, 108
Witch hazel, 185
Wrinkles, herbal remedies for, 262–263
Wu Shi Er Bing Fang (Prescriptions for Fifty-two Diseases), 29, 190

Yeast infections, herbs for, 231–232
Ye Ju, 193
Yerba santa, 166–167
Yin and yang, 191
Yucca, 167–168

Zimu, 192